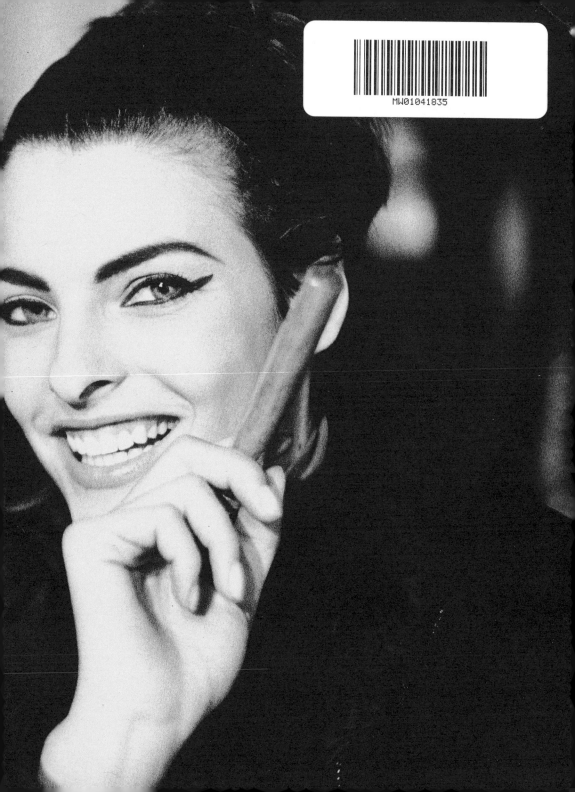

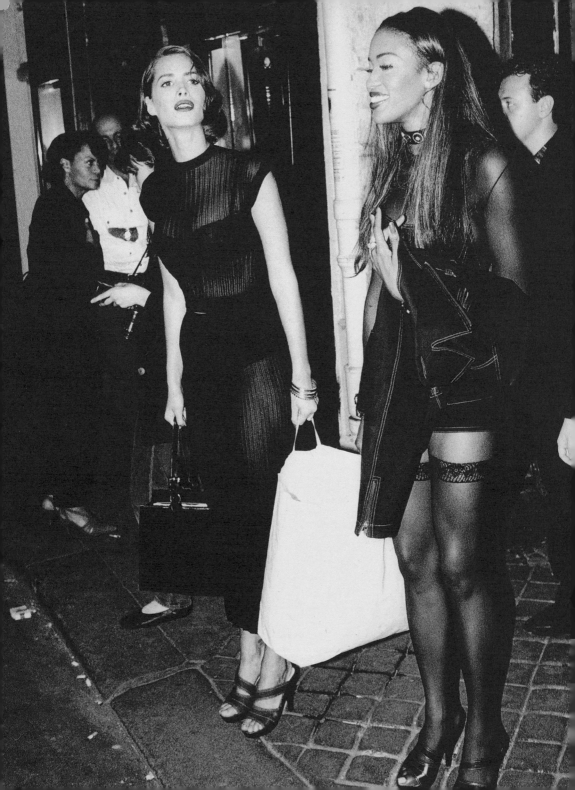

ARTHUR ELGORT'S MODELS MANUAL

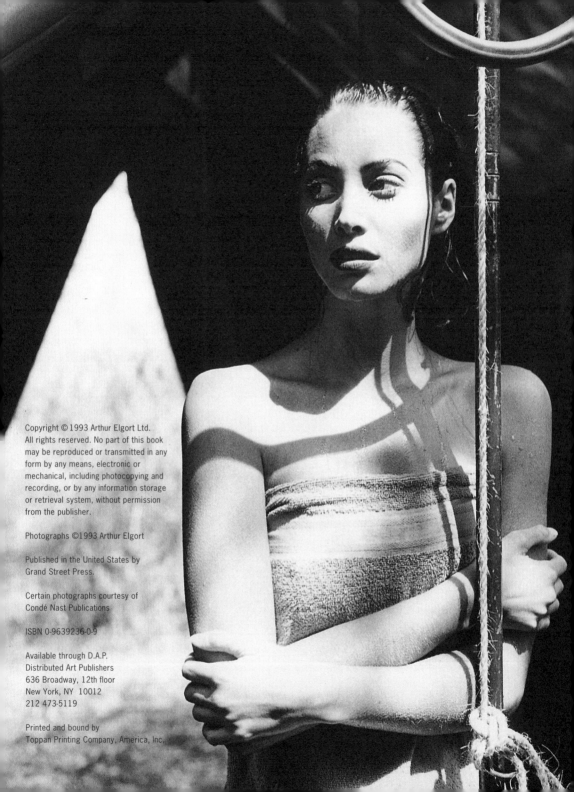

Photographs ©1993 Arthur Elgort

Published in the United States by
Grand Street Press.

Certain photographs courtesy of
Condé Nast Publications

ISBN 0-9639236-0-9

Available through D.A.P.
Distributed Art Publishers
636 Broadway, 12th floor
New York, NY 10012
212 473-5119

Printed and bound by
Toppan Printing Company, America, Inc.

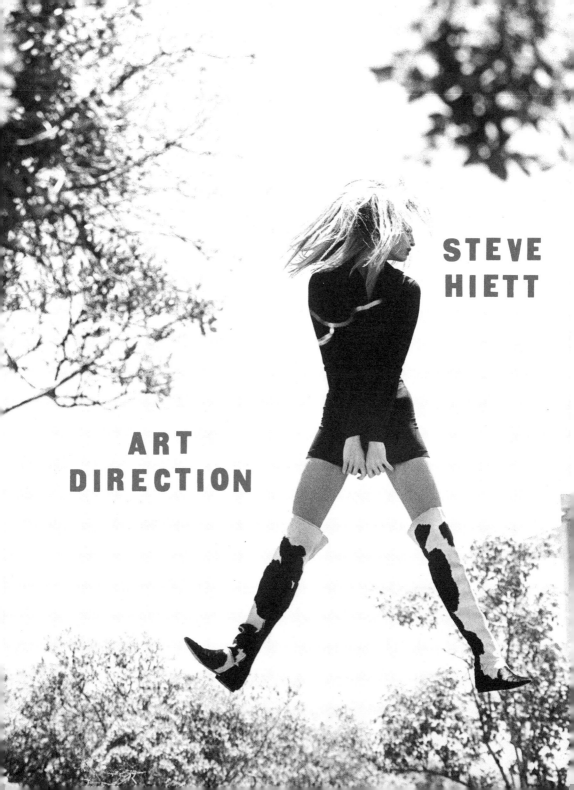

STEVE
HIETT

ART
DIRECTION

This book is a tribute
to alot of the models I
have photographed, with
a look at some unique
individuals in my fashion
life.

Arthur Elgort

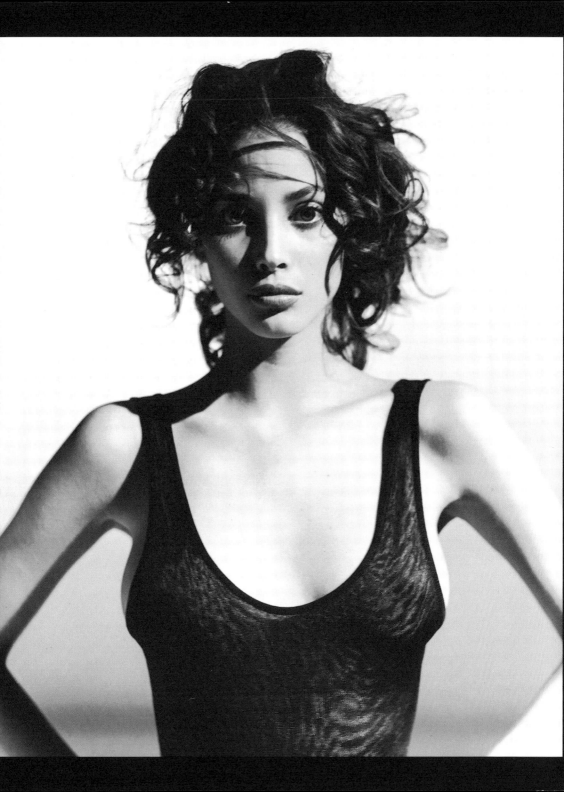

L/NDA

EVANGELISTA

"I started
right at the bottom. I
entered a contest to be
'Miss Teen Canada,' and I
didn't even place. I was sixteen. I
finished school six months early and
went to New York. I saw every photographer. None wanted to work with me,
no one wanted to test me. My mother
had to send me money so that I could
pay for test shots. A month later, I went
to Paris and Elite threw out all the shots I
had paid to have done. I did 'mini' editorial for minor magazines. But that's
not what I wanted to do. I never got
frustrated, because I thought that
was the way it was. I didn't
think you could just
start at the top."

Linda showed up one day at my hotel in
Paris. She was sassy and smart and remind-
ed me of Joan Severance. She had that look
that said, "I know I'm going to be fabu-
lous—you give me a chance."

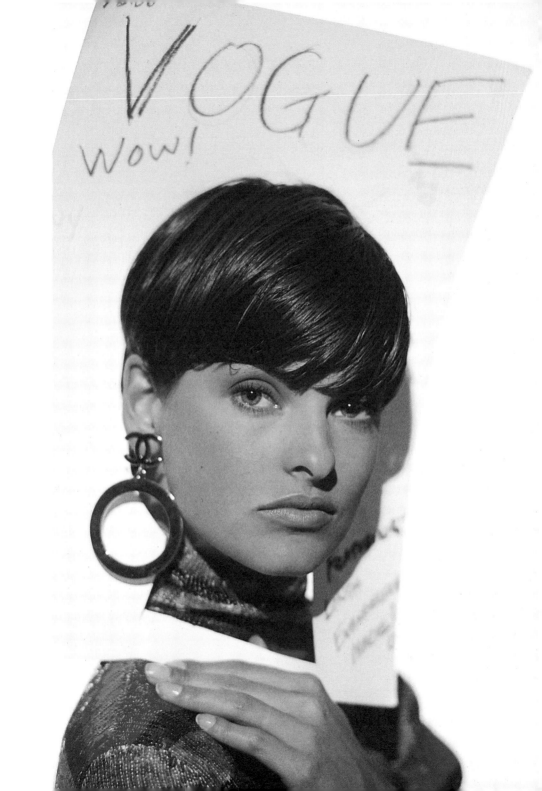

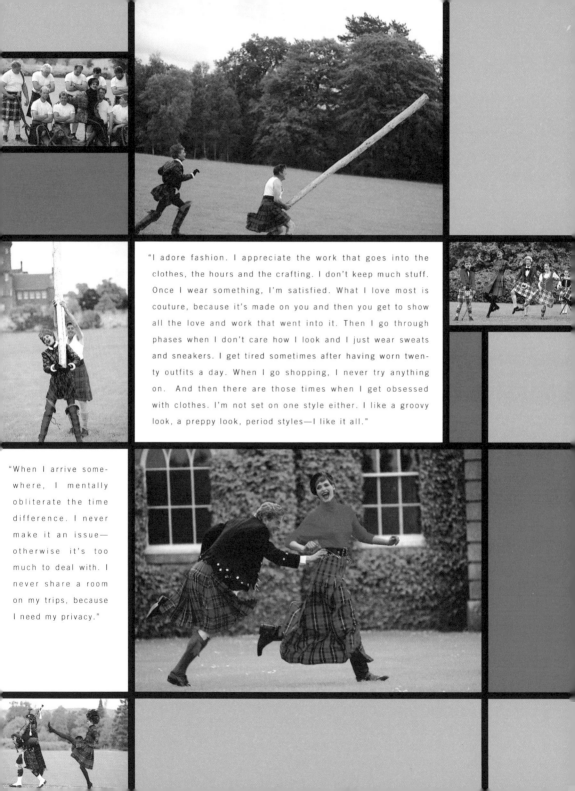

"I adore fashion. I appreciate the work that goes into the clothes, the hours and the crafting. I don't keep much stuff. Once I wear something, I'm satisfied. What I love most is couture, because it's made on you and then you get to show all the love and work that went into it. Then I go through phases when I don't care how I look and I just wear sweats and sneakers. I get tired sometimes after having worn twenty outfits a day. When I go shopping, I never try anything on. And then there are those times when I get obsessed with clothes. I'm not set on one style either. I like a groovy look, a preppy look, period styles—I like it all."

"When I arrive some-where, I mentally obliterate the time difference. I never make it an issue—otherwise it's too much to deal with. I never share a room on my trips, because I need my privacy."

"I ALWAYS WANTED TO BE A MODEL. I WASN'T THINK-ING ABOUT THE TRAVEL-ING, THE GLAMOUR, THE MONEY...NONE OF THAT. I JUST WANTED TO WEAR THE BEST FASHIONS IN THE BEST PHOTOGRAPHS. I HAVE THE DRIVE FOR IT."

"I started on a very commercial path, but no one, thankfully, noticed. By the time I was recommended to *Vogue* and all those other magazines, I had figured out who was who and what was what. I bought every single magazine and looked at every page. Agencies can't tell you everything. You have to find out on your own."

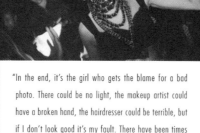

"In the end, it's the girl who gets the blame for a bad photo. There could be no light, the makeup artist could have a broken hand, the hairdresser could be terrible, but if I don't look good it's my fault. There have been times when I wanted to buy every issue of a magazine off the newsstands. I have a whole archive of what I call my 'doozies.'"

"A model is dependent on many different professionals. You can't be one without an agent, without photographers. I've learned to put all my cards on the table, and I arrange them the way I want them. I make all my own decisions."

"I never walk out on a job. When things get bad with a particular client, I say to myself, 'Where am I going from here? What else would I rather be doing?' There is no other job that can beat this."

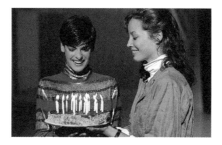

"I don't diet. I just don't eat as much as I'd like to."

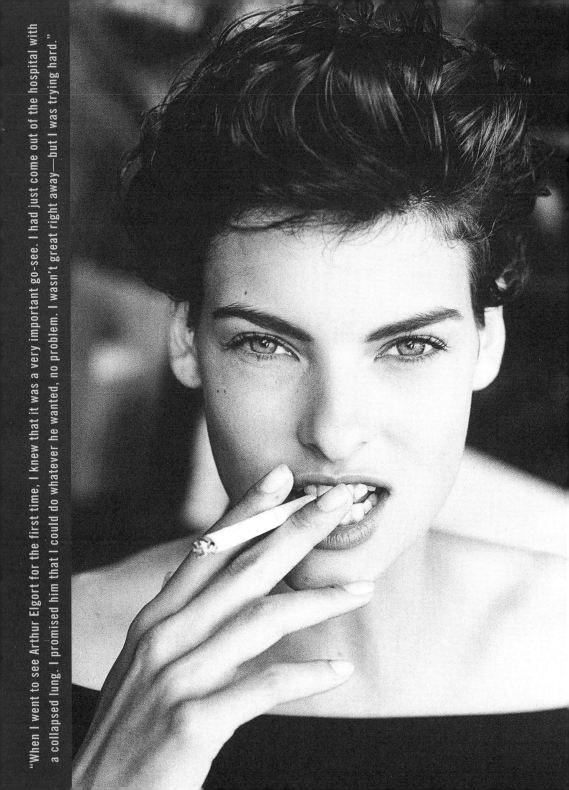

"When I went to see Arthur Elgort for the first time, I knew that it was a very important go-see. I had just come out of the hospital with a collapsed lung. I promised him that I could do whatever he wanted, no problem. I wasn't great right away—but I was trying hard."

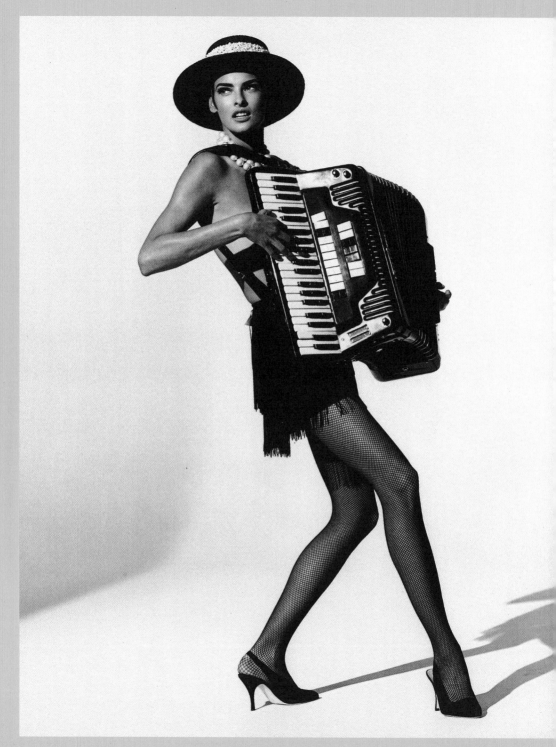

Linda's got nerve and the body to back it up – gorgeous knees and ankles. She really can play the accord

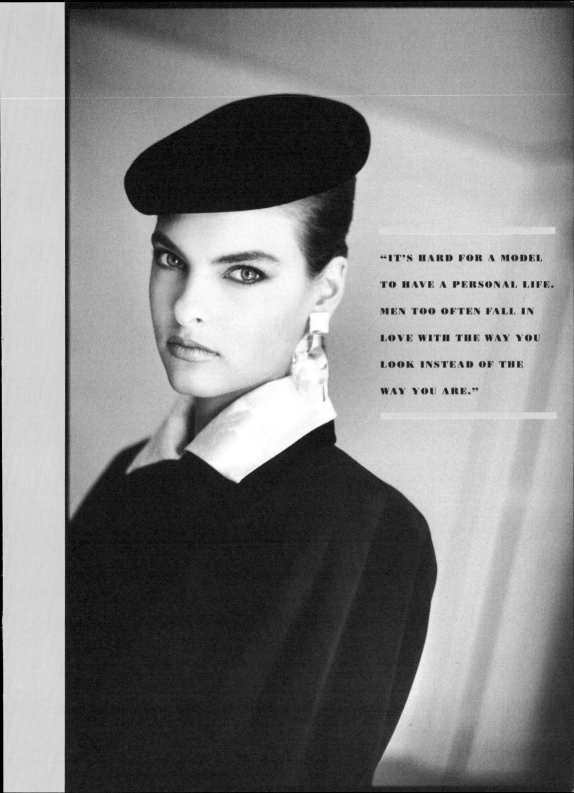

"IT'S HARD FOR A MODEL TO HAVE A PERSONAL LIFE. MEN TOO OFTEN FALL IN LOVE WITH THE WAY YOU LOOK INSTEAD OF THE WAY YOU ARE."

"What about the future? I used to say I don't know. There are so many doors open to me now. I want to do something that I enjoy as much as this. It doesn't have to be as financially rewarding—I just want to enjoy it. I wasn't put on this earth to be a model. This is just a passing thing."

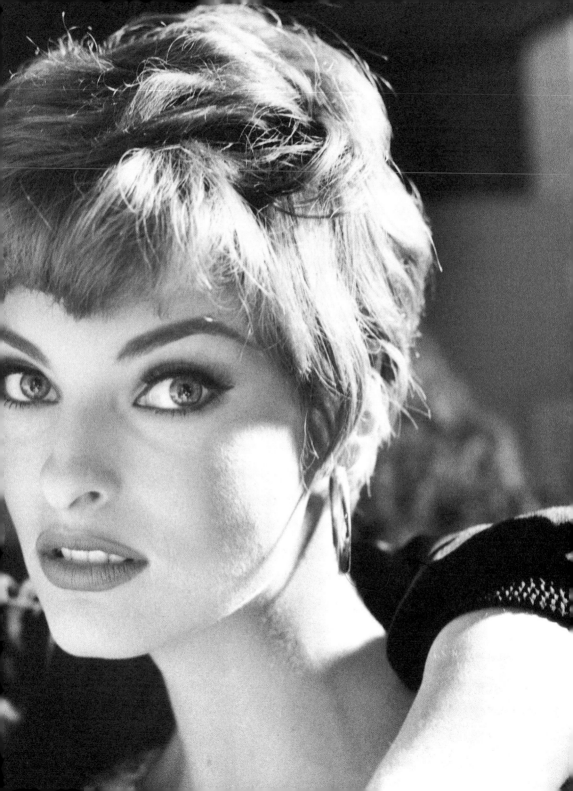

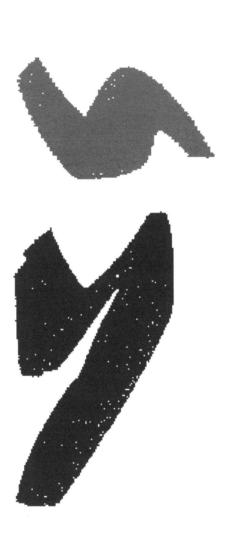

susan holmes

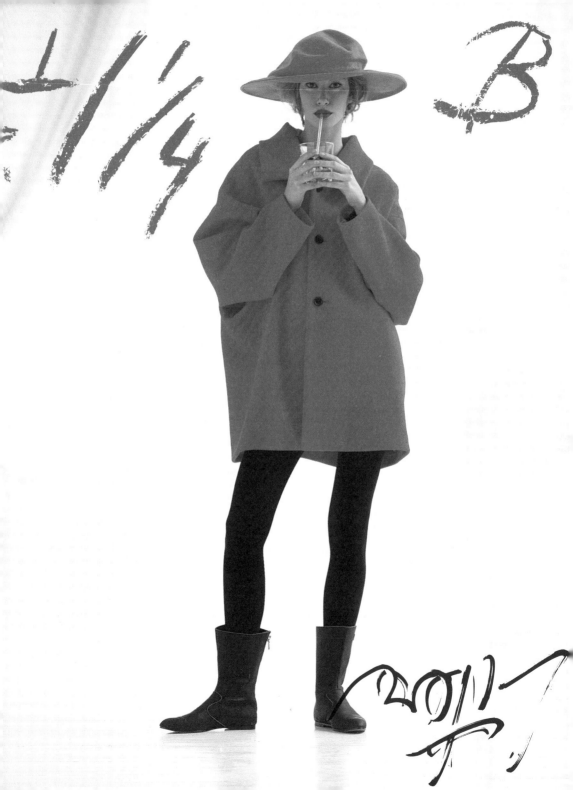

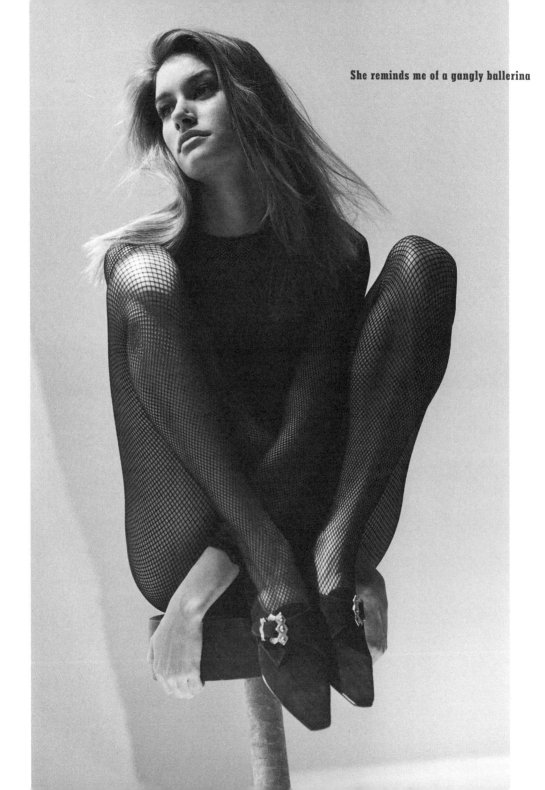

She reminds me of a gangly ballerina

HOW I GOT MY START I WAS ALWAYS INTERESTED IN MODELING. MY FIRST TEST SHOTS WERE IN SAN DIEGO, WHEN I WAS SIXTEEN. MY MOM DIDN'T WANT ME TO MODEL, SO I FINISHED HIGH SCHOOL—I'M REALLY GLAD I DID.

MY FIRST JOB I WORKED IN A PIZZA PARLOR AS A DISHWASHER.

MY MOST EMBARRASSING MOMENT WHEN I WAS WORKING ON A SHOOT IN TAHITI, THERE WERE SAILORS WITH ME IN THE PHOTOGRAPH AND THEY MISUNDERSTOOD THE PHOTOGRAPHER'S DIRECTIONS. AFTER TWO HOURS OF ELAB-ORATE HAIR AND MAKEUP, THEY THREW ME INTO THE OCEAN—MANOLO BLAHNIKS AND ALL.

WHEN MODELING IS BORING DOING CATALOGUES.

THE DOWN SIDE OF MODELING WITH TRAVELING TWO TO THREE WEEKS EVERY MONTH IT'S REALLY A GYPSY LIFE-STYLE, SOMETIMES YOU JUST WANT TO STAY HOME.

REGRETS IT TOOK ME A LONG TIME TO LEARN TO GO WITH MY INSTINCTS. IN THE BEGINNING, AN AGENT WILL SEND YOU ANYWHERE—UNTIL YOU SAY NO, YOU ARE NOT YOUR OWN BOSS.

CHILDHOOD DREAM: UNTIL I WAS EIGHT, I WANTED TO BE AN OLYMPIC ICE SKATER. NOW I NEVER HAVE TIME TO SKATE.

WHAT I DO WHEN I'M NOT WORKING SLEEP, SEE FRIENDS AND GO TO MOVIES. I LOVE TO HEAR LIVE MUSIC, I GUESS YOU'D SAY I'M A PARTIER.

WHAT I THINK ABOUT MY LOOKS I THINK I HAVE A STRANGE LOOK. MY WORST FEATURE IS MY EARS—I ALWAYS HAVE TO ASK THE HAIRDRESSER TO COVER THEM.

FAVORITE CLOTHES I LOVE SHOPPING THE THRIFT STORES. I JUST BOUGHT A PAIR OF GOLD SANDALS FROM THE SEVENTIES FOR $1.99 AND A GREEN VELVET DRESS MADE IN PARIS FOR $50. MY FAVORITE FIND-OF-THE-MOMENT IS A BROWN FAKE FUZZY FUR JACKET WITH RED QUILTED LINING THAT COST ALMOST NOTHING.

WHAT I PACK FOR A TWO-DAY TRIP BLUE JEANS, WHITE T-SHIRTS AND BLACK SUEDE LACE-UP JEANS WITH PATENT-LEATHER MOTORCYCLE BOOTS.

FAVORITE MUSIC DYLAN, THE STONES, JANIS JOPLIN, ALTERNATIVE MUSIC.

MY NIGHT OWL UNIFORM BLACK VELVET BELL-BOTTOMS, A POLYESTER SHIRT IN A FUNNY PRINT, CHOKER AND CHAINS.

WHAT I THINK ABOUT THE SIXTIES REVIVAL IT'S A RELIEF TO GET OUT OF THE YUPPIE SCENE.

WHAT I DO WHEN I STAY HOME, WHICH IS RARE THIS IS THE FIRST TIME I HAVE AN APARTMENT OF MY OWN. I'VE LIVED IN PARIS FOR TWO AND A HALF YEARS, SO I'M LEARNING TO COOK.

FAVORITE FOOD SUSHI, PIZZA.

FAVORITE HOTEL 29 PALMS INN.

WHAT I KEEP ON MY BEDSIDE TABLE A BOX OF HOT TAMALES (I DON'T HAVE THEM RIGHT NOW BECAUSE I ATE THEM ALL) AND BOOKS. I JUST FINISHED TOM ROBBINS'S *SKINNY LEGS AND ALL* AND THE WARHOL BIOGRAPHY.

WHAT I DO WITH MY MONEY MY MOM HELPS ME.

WHAT I WOULD CHANGE IF I COULD I WISH I WERE SHORTER SO I COULD WEAR HIGH HEELS AND NOT TOWER OVER MEN.

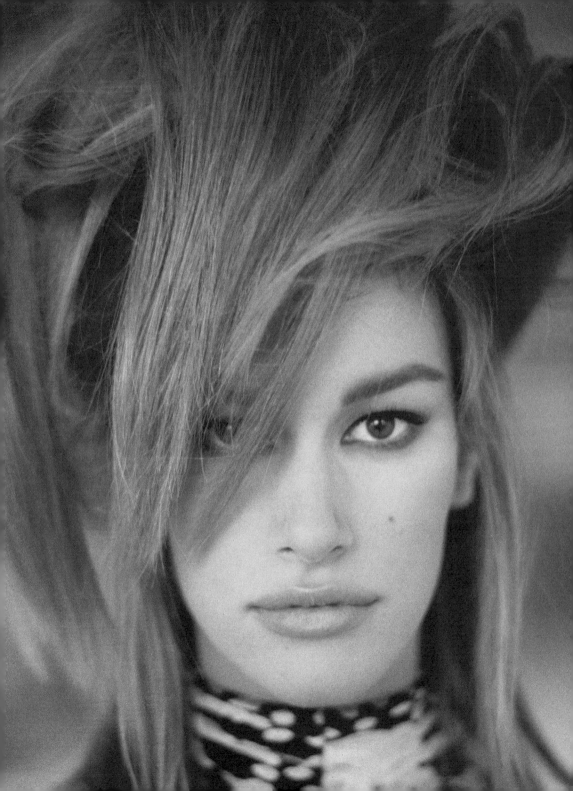

She's always into it – disciplined, funny and the legs to go with it

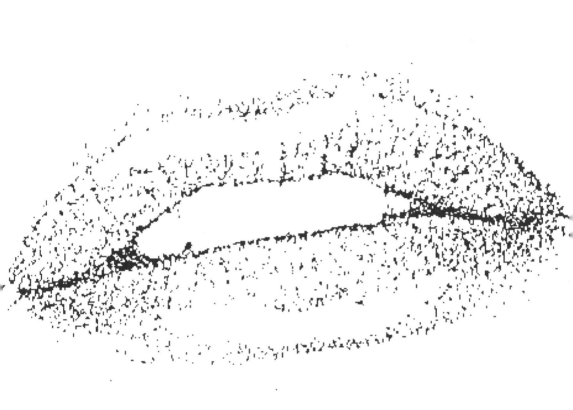

"I get sick of makeup"

There's nothing like humor with some good looks attached to it

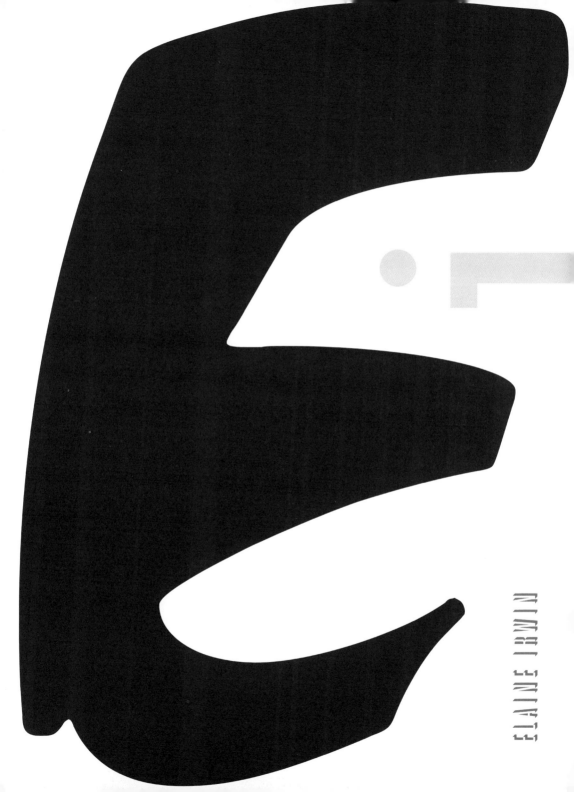

ELAINE IRWIN

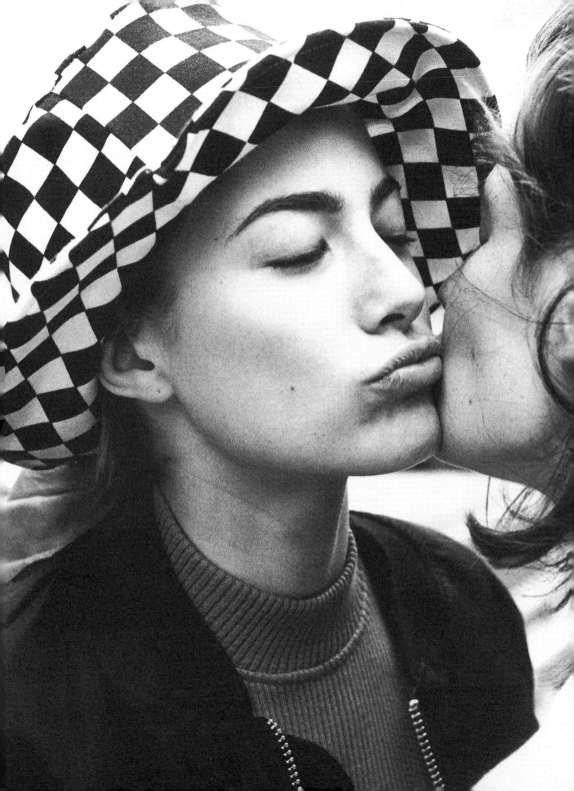

How did you get your start?

I stumbled into it. I was eighteen, when by accident I met the president of Elite. Afterward, that trip to New York City was really my first time there as an adult. I'd never been on the twenty-sixth floor of a skyscraper before.

What was your first shoot like?

It was for *Seventeen* magazine. I remember being thrilled—even when the photo came out in the magazine the size of a postage stamp.

What was the most embarrassing thing that ever happened on a shoot?

I got hit by a bus on the way to my first big European photo shoot in London.

Any advice to beginners?

It's easy to take things personally, especially when you're starting out. Maybe a photographer will change his mind about you or something. But you can't let it get to you or let it take over your life.

Before you fell into modeling, what were your dreams for the future?

I had finished high school and wanted to be a chemical engineer, a toxicologist actually. I wanted to help save the environment.

What did you do with your down time when you weren't modeling?

What down time?

When you were living in your New York apartment, what was in your refrigerator?

It was empty. I was not much of a cook—it was a disgrace.

What do you think photographers saw in you?

Who knows? Well, I guess my eyes are nice to photograph, as long as they don't look too squinty.

Any jobs before modeling?

I counted nails in a hardware store.

What are you doing now?

I've started to shift priorities. I'm married and live in Indianapolis, Indiana, where my husband is from. I'm now a stepmother and a grandmother at twenty-three. We live in a big house in the woods. I have a dog, a Siamese cat, two horses, a pig, two mice and a rat. I bought the rat in New York—really, it's an easy pet to take care of.

Future plans?

I want to learn how to paint and sculpt.

TO SMILE...

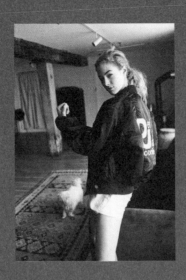

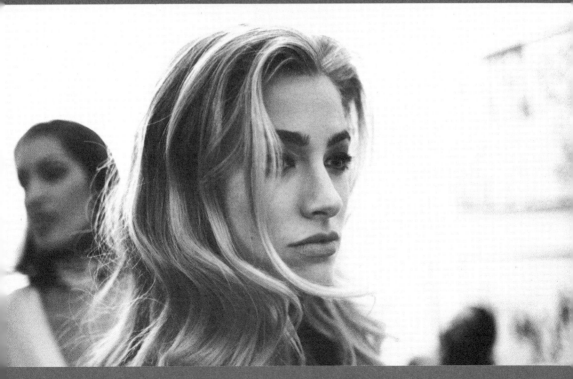

EEL LIKE IT."

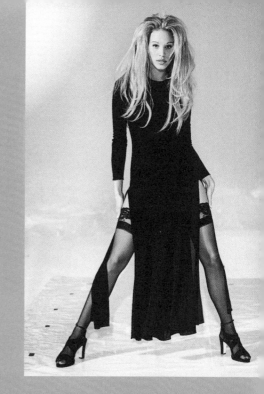

"I'M

NOT

A GLAMOUR MODEL..........

I'm more the sporty, tomboy type."......

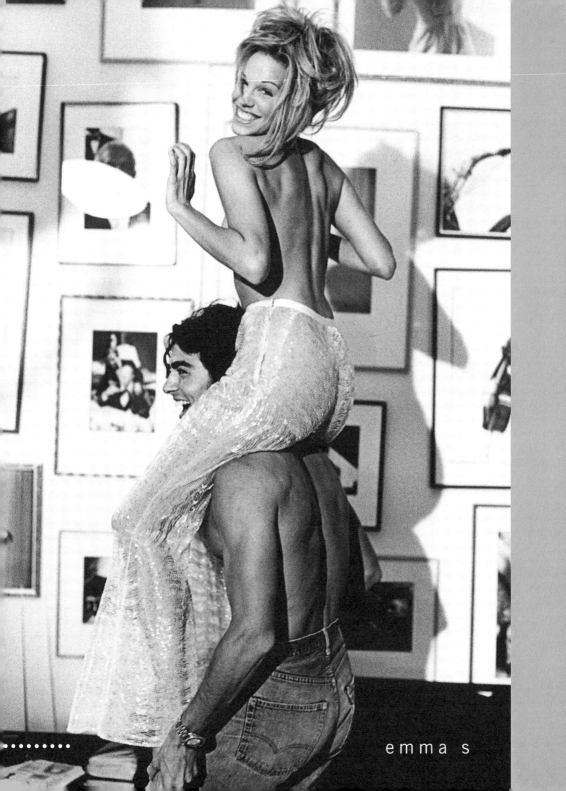

emma s

A PERFECT EXAMPLE OF A GOOD GO SEE. SHE IS READY TO HAVE HER PICTURE TAKEN AND JUMP!

remember my first go-see with Arthur. It was a very, very hot day and so I was earing a little white dress. I had no makeup on. I was the last girl to show up. rst we talked, and then Arthur started smoking his pipe. He had his trumpet with m and I asked him to play, and next thing I knew I was jumping around on the sofa. Arthur always has his camera around his neck, so he started snapping. I danced for ten years before I started modeling, so it just sort of came naturally.

Those pictures he took have always been among my favorites....

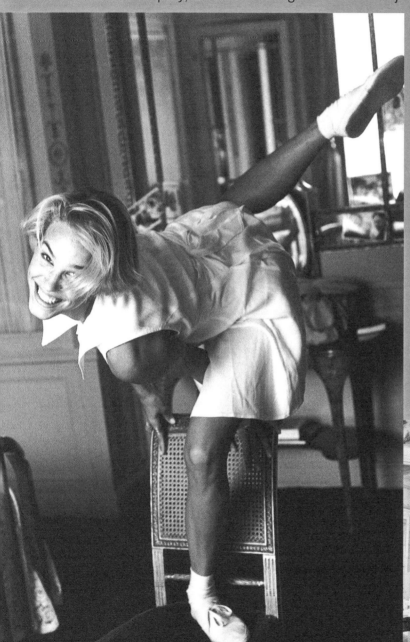

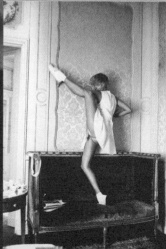

paulina

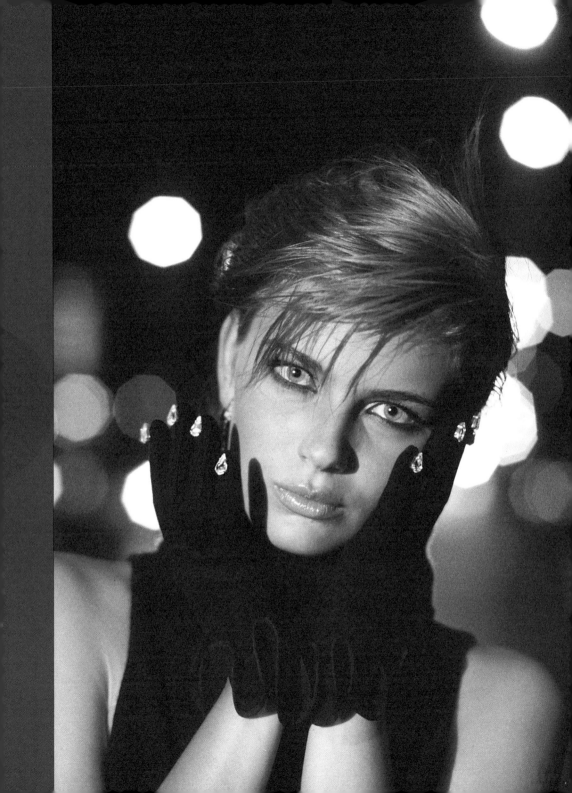

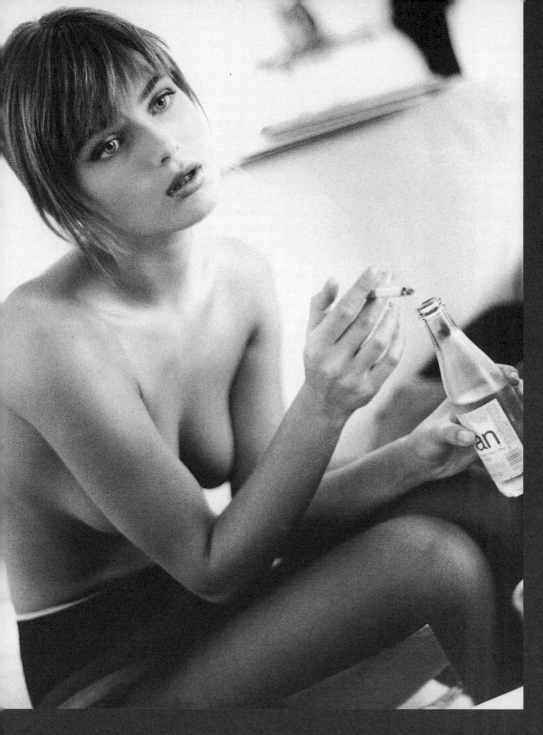

"I'm too European to live in California—I like cigarette smoke too much."

She never changed her look. It was always, "I'm Pauline. I am what I am."

"I was 15 when I first shot with Arthur for Chanel in Paris."

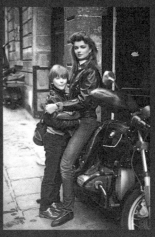

"I felt like a naive little idiot. I was intimidated and scared."

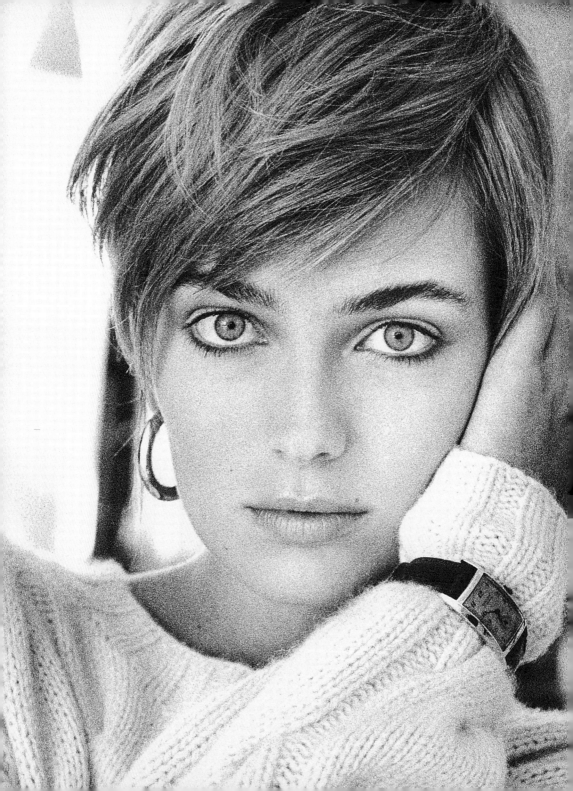

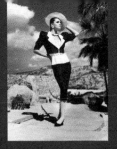

Money makes the shit we go through all worthwhile. ● How did I handle rejection? When you're 15, it hurts a lot. ● I always had a hang-up about being thought stupid because I was a model, but I knew differently. I always read, paint, and I play classical music. ● I guess a part of me was always trying to rebel against an image. I always shopped at Trash and Vaudeville, carried a pack of Marlboro and swore. I liked looking like I

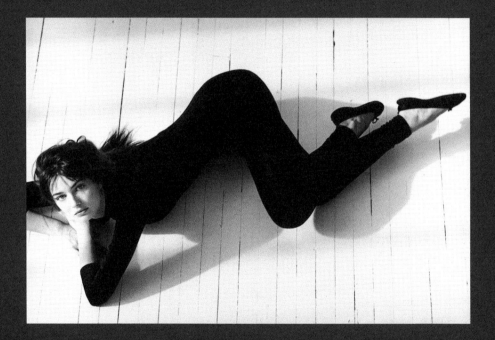

"There's plenty of stress, but there are also those little glamorous moments when you eel pretty and you know you're getting a great picture."

walked out of a B-movie. ● I have never exercised in my life. ● I believed I was totally plain, if not on the ugly side. I've felt like an imposter the whole way. I was always grateful for anyone who thought I was attractive. ● I've always wanted to dye my hair black. ● The photographer is the director. A really good model makes it look so easy. ● I never wake up and say to myself in the mirror, "you look pretty"— all I see are the bags under my eyes. That's where the hair-and-makeup artists come in, they're the miracle workers. ● Future plans? I want to learn to play the harp and speak Chinese.

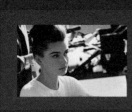

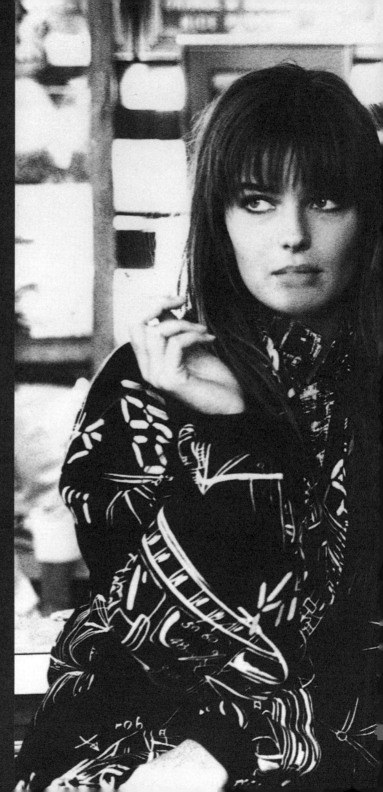

"I fell in love instantly—it was all physical. I knew when I first laid eyes on Ric that he was the man of my dreams and that I was going to marry him."

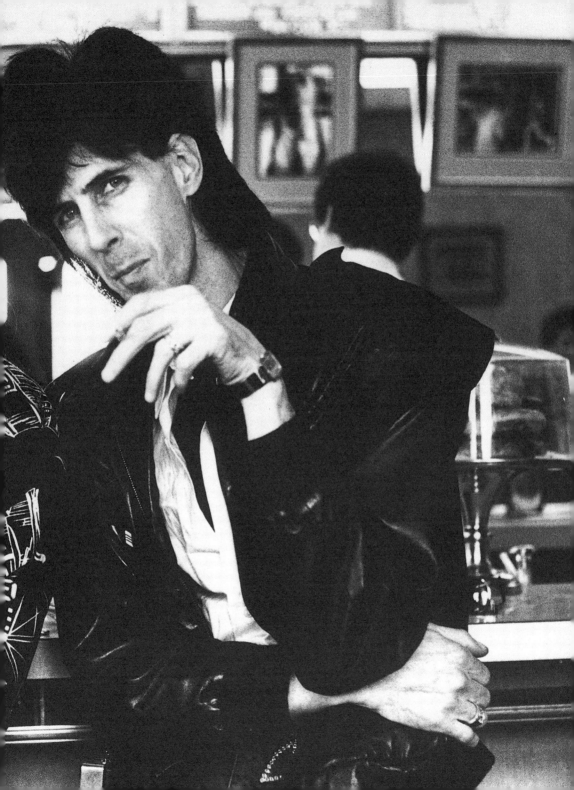

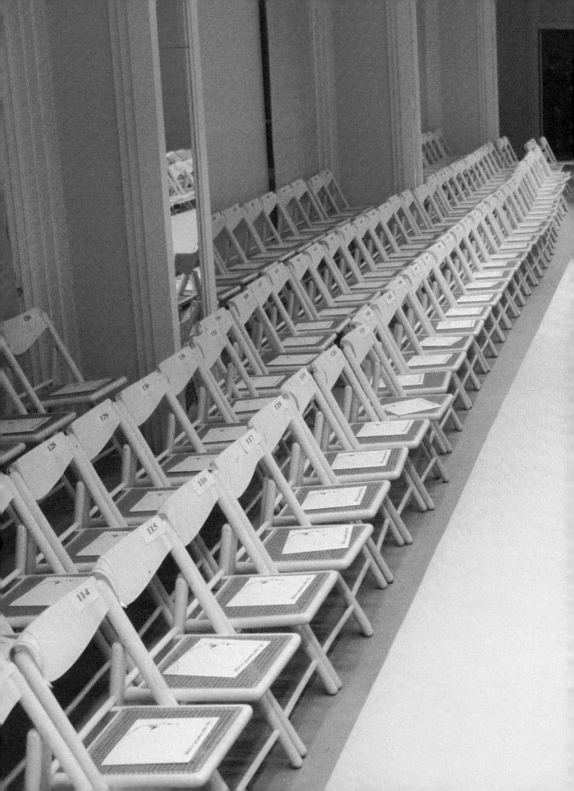

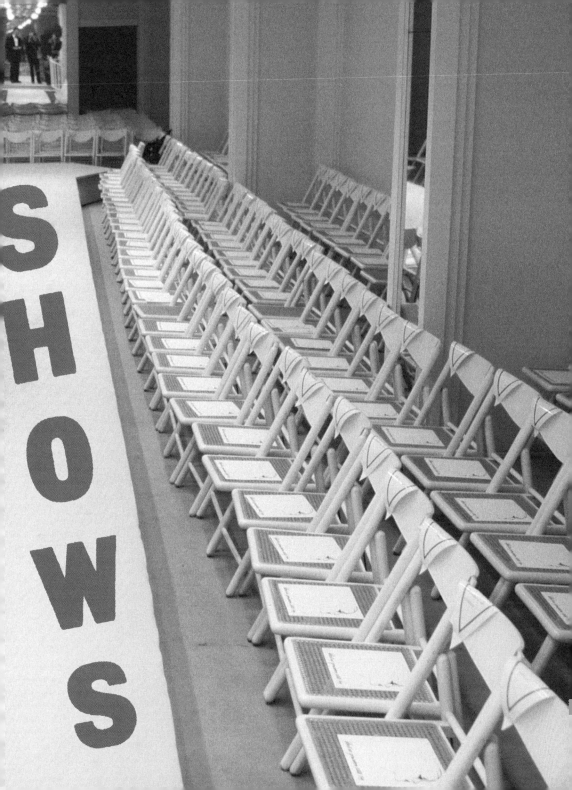

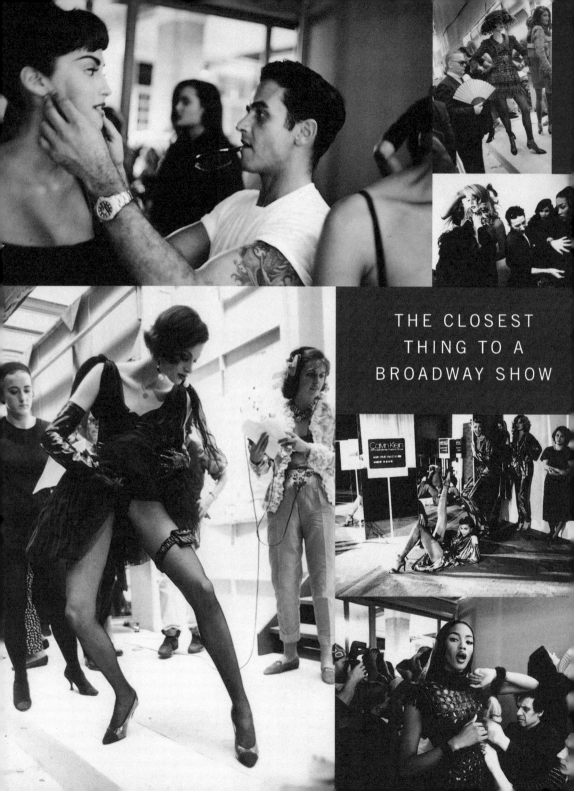

THE CLOSEST
THING TO A
BROADWAY SHOW

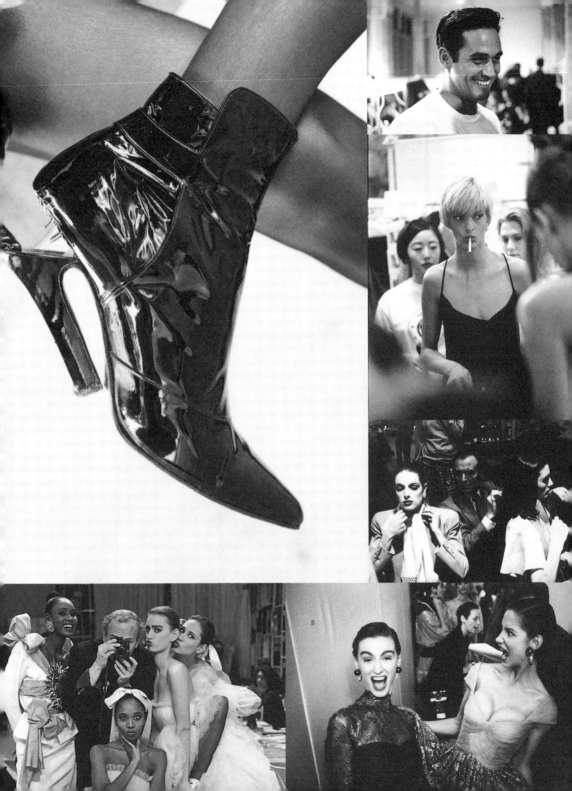

CHECKING
TO SEE
WHO'S ARRIVED...
IS AMERICAN
VOGUE HERE?

Can we begin!

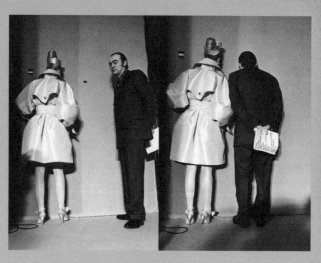

CHRISTIAN LACROIX AND MARIE

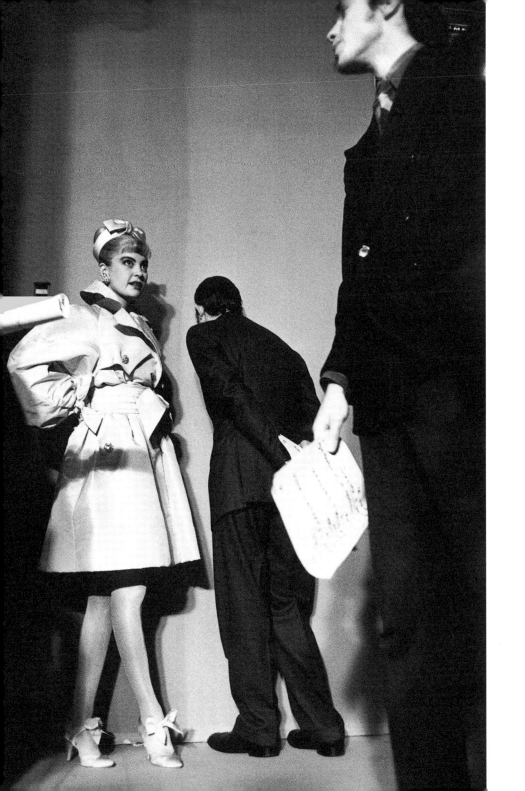

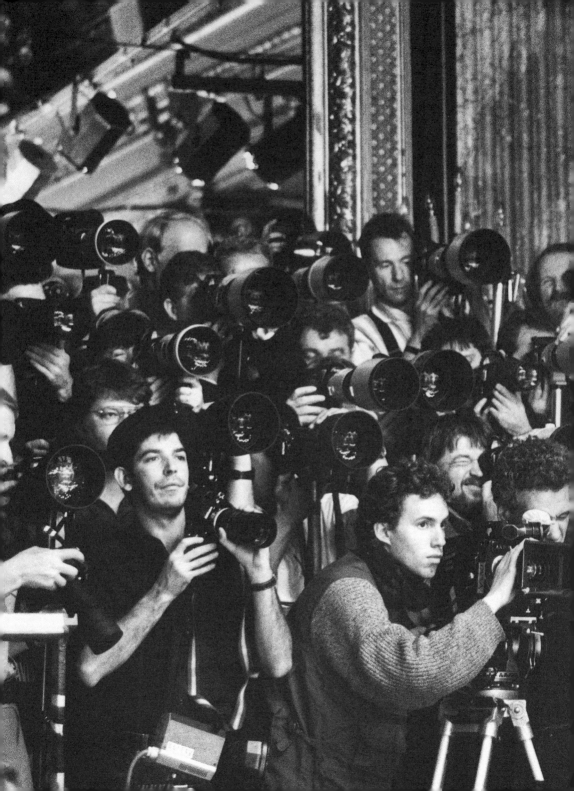

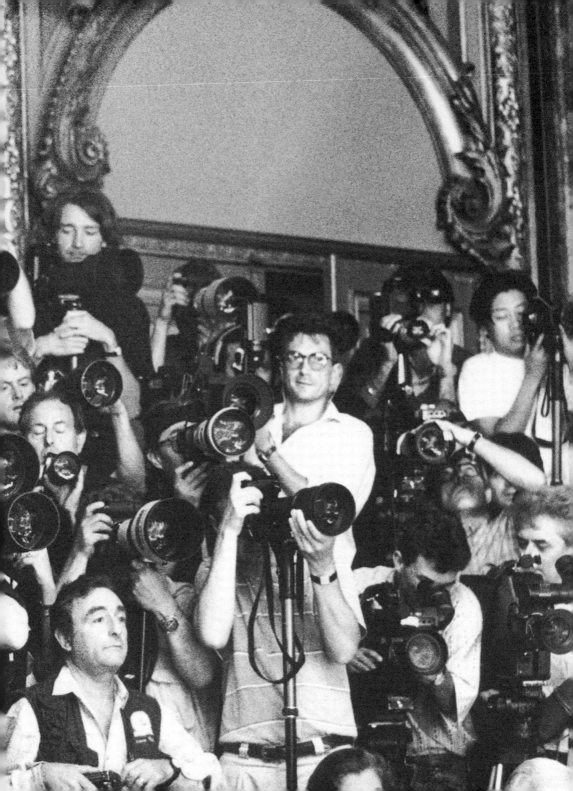

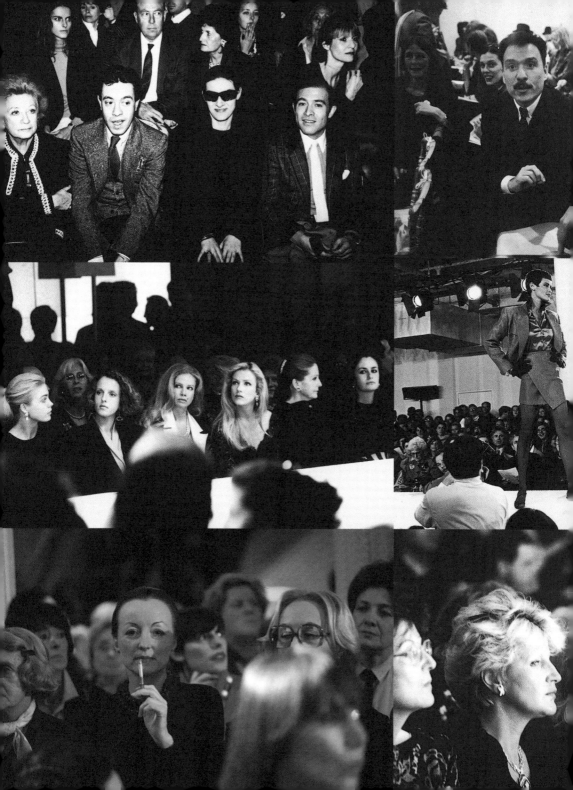

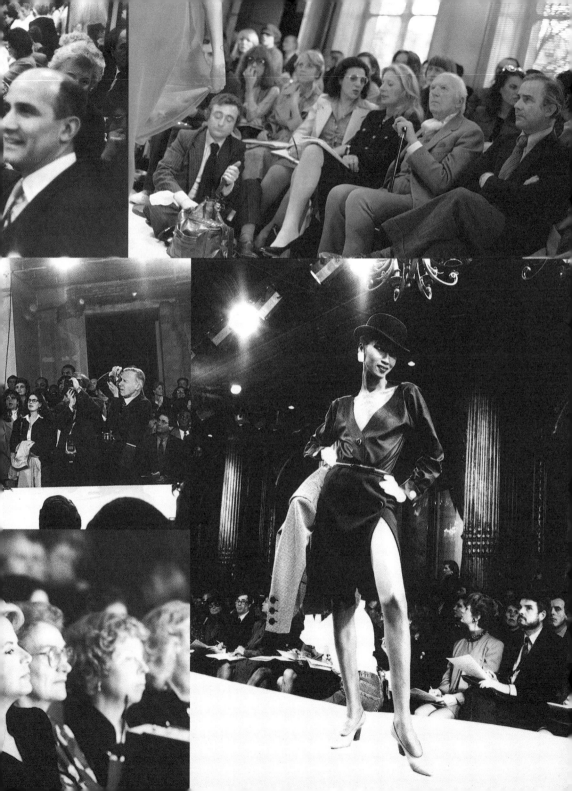

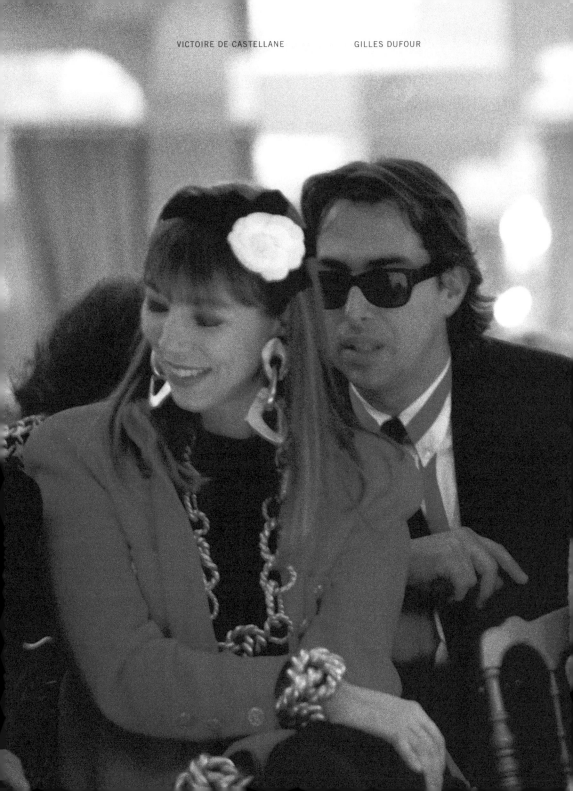

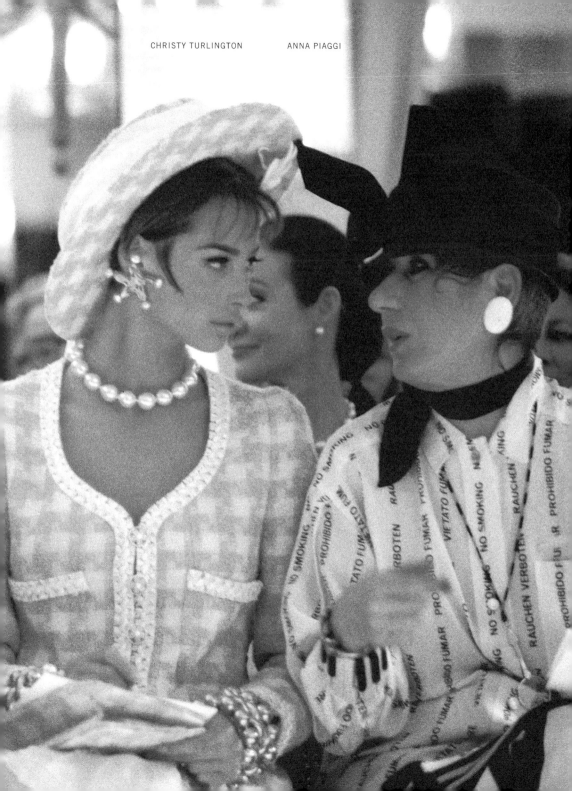

SCAR

IT

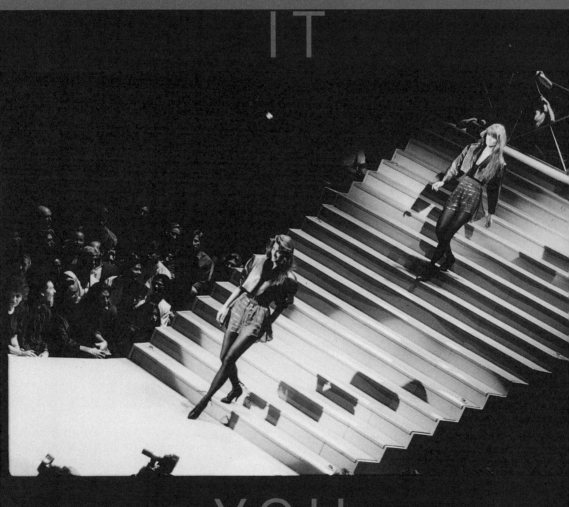

YOU

FALL

ED OF

MAKES

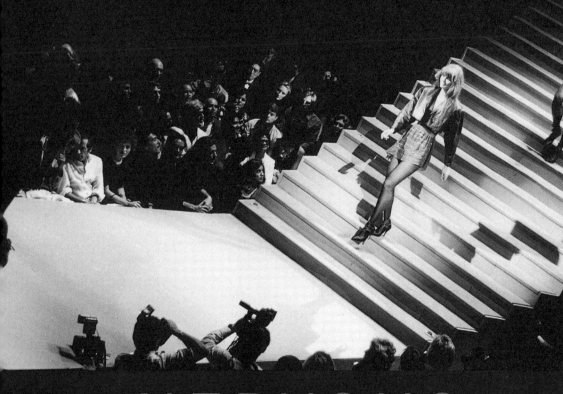

NERVOUS

ING!

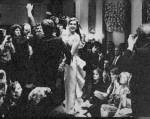

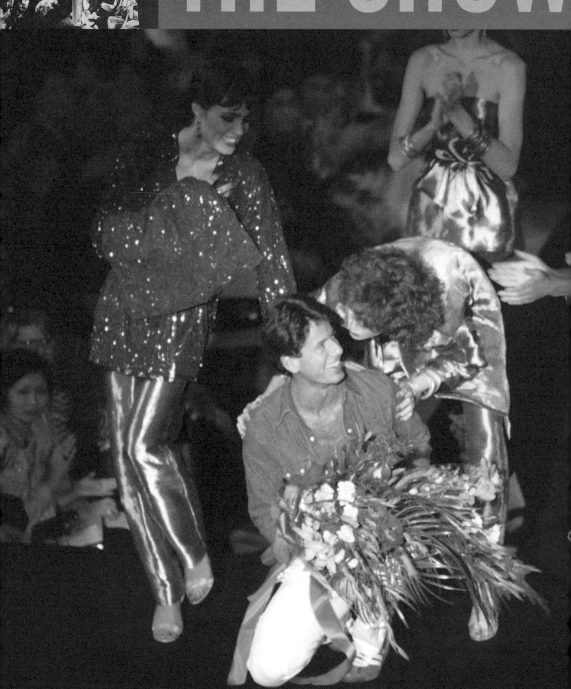

IS OVER.......!

Relief! Run to the next!

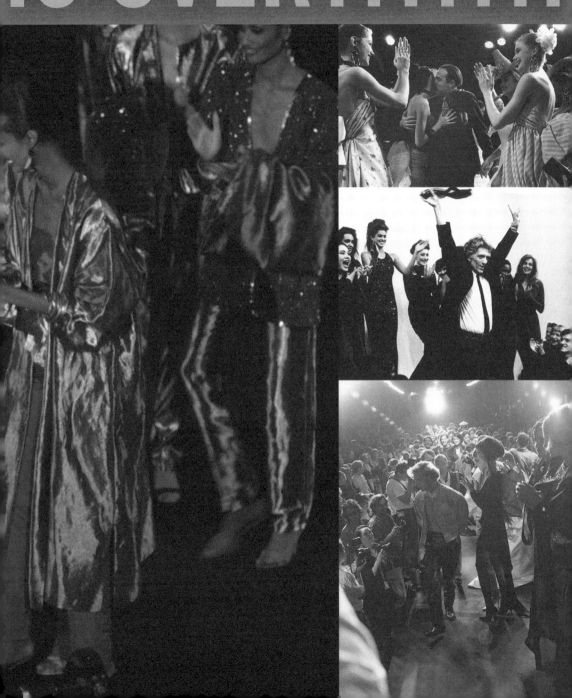

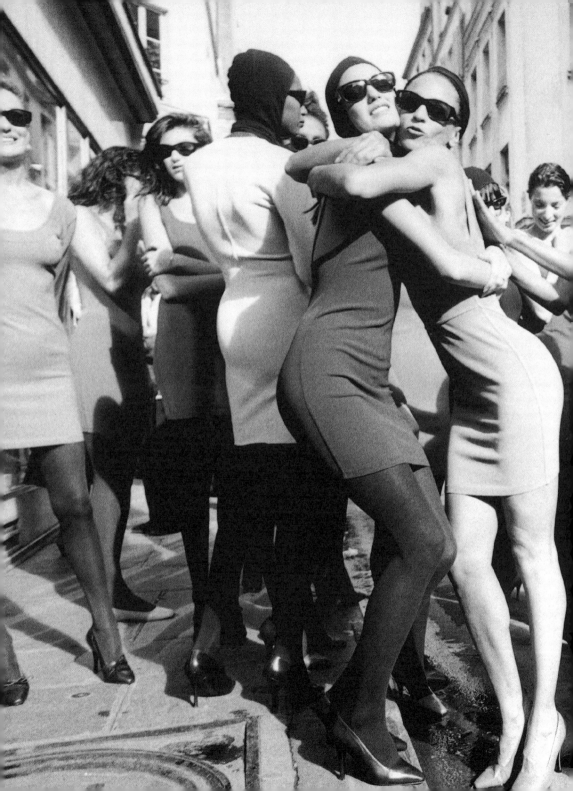

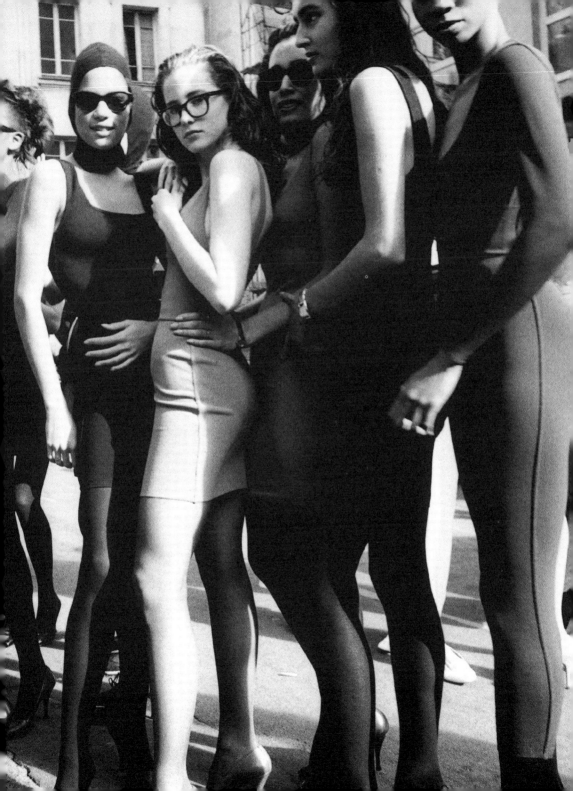

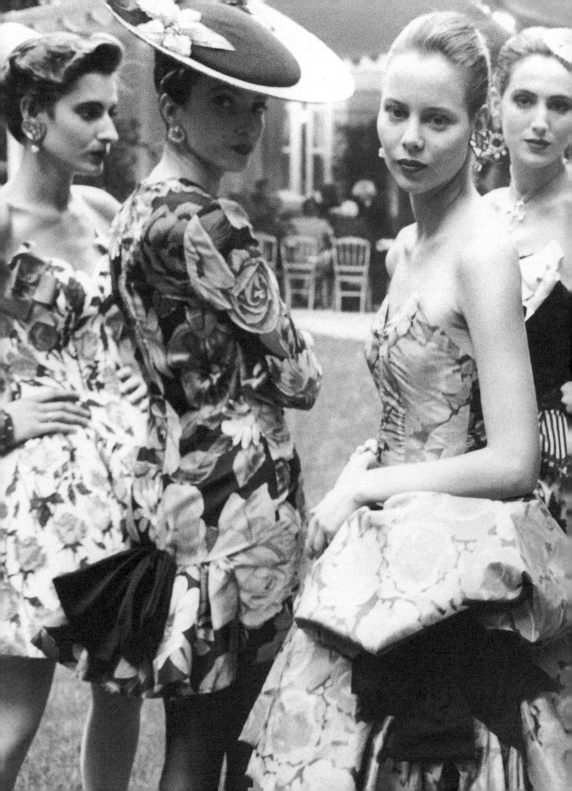

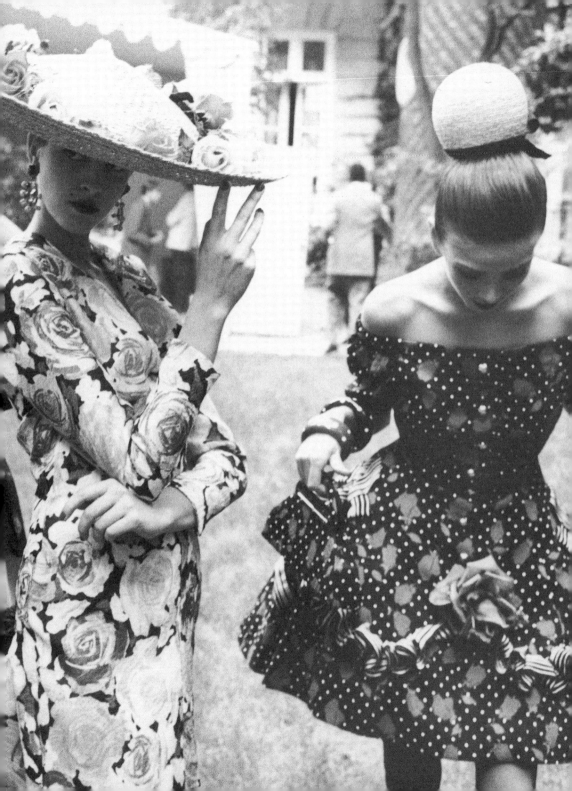

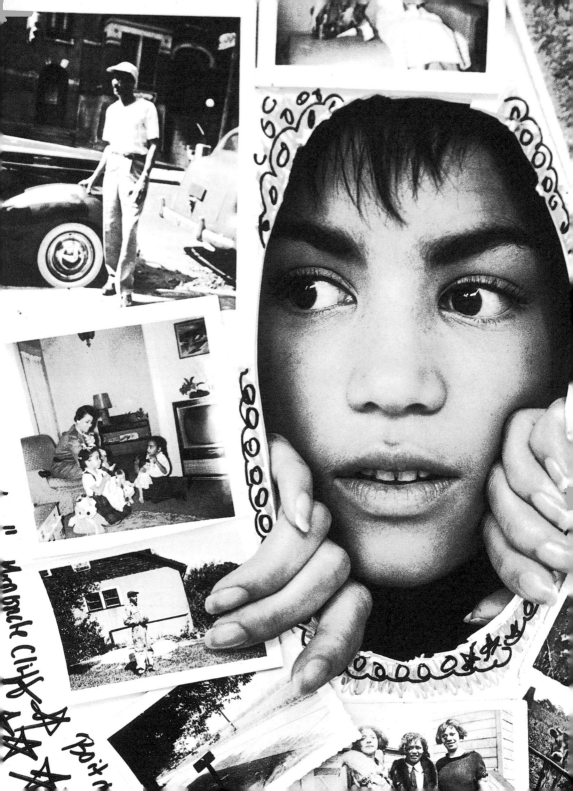

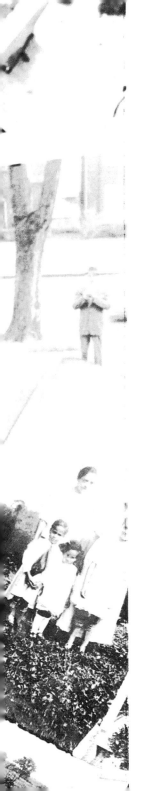
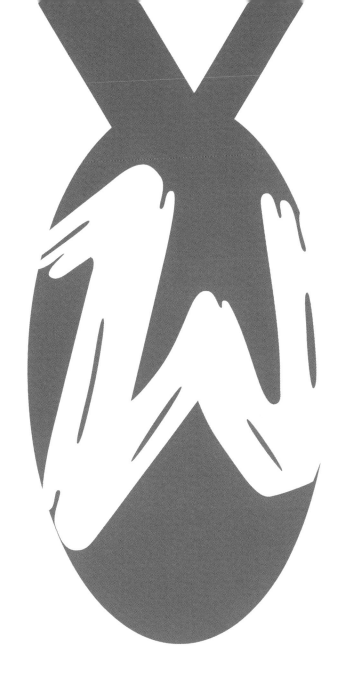

VERONICA WEBB

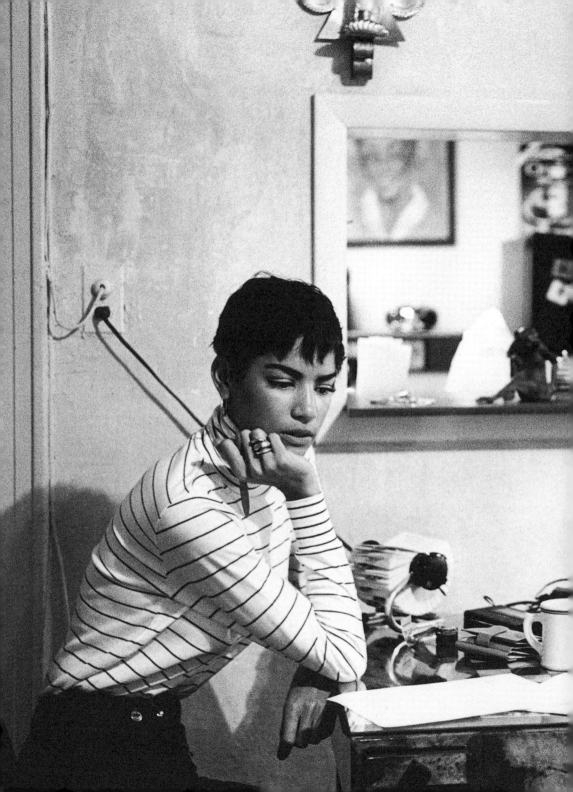

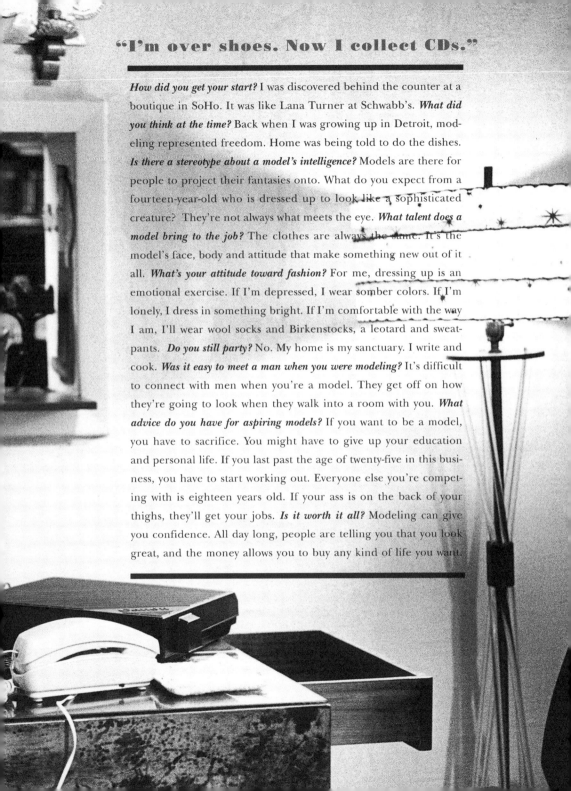

"I'm over shoes. Now I collect CDs."

How did you get your start? I was discovered behind the counter at a boutique in SoHo. It was like Lana Turner at Schwabb's. *What did you think at the time?* Back when I was growing up in Detroit, modeling represented freedom. Home was being told to do the dishes. *Is there a stereotype about a model's intelligence?* Models are there for people to project their fantasies onto. What do you expect from a fourteen-year-old who is dressed up to look like a sophisticated creature? They're not always what meets the eye. *What talent does a model bring to the job?* The clothes are always the same. It's the model's face, body and attitude that make something new out of it all. *What's your attitude toward fashion?* For me, dressing up is an emotional exercise. If I'm depressed, I wear somber colors. If I'm lonely, I dress in something bright. If I'm comfortable with the way I am, I'll wear wool socks and Birkenstocks, a leotard and sweatpants. *Do you still party?* No. My home is my sanctuary. I write and cook. *Was it easy to meet a man when you were modeling?* It's difficult to connect with men when you're a model. They get off on how they're going to look when they walk into a room with you. *What advice do you have for aspiring models?* If you want to be a model, you have to sacrifice. You might have to give up your education and personal life. If you last past the age of twenty-five in this business, you have to start working out. Everyone else you're competing with is eighteen years old. If your ass is on the back of your thighs, they'll get your jobs. *Is it worth it all?* Modeling can give you confidence. All day long, people are telling you that you look great, and the money allows you to buy any kind of life you want.

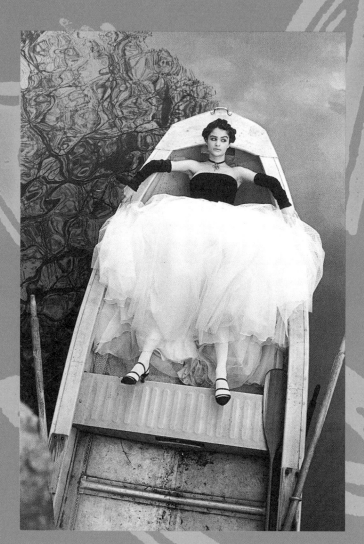

"I'm from Denmark. Nobody cares that I'm a model back home."

HELENA CHRISTENSEN

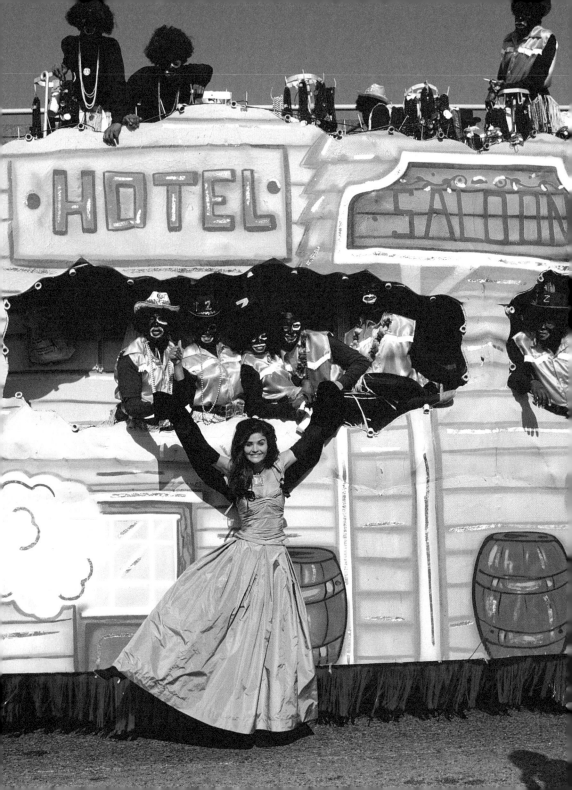

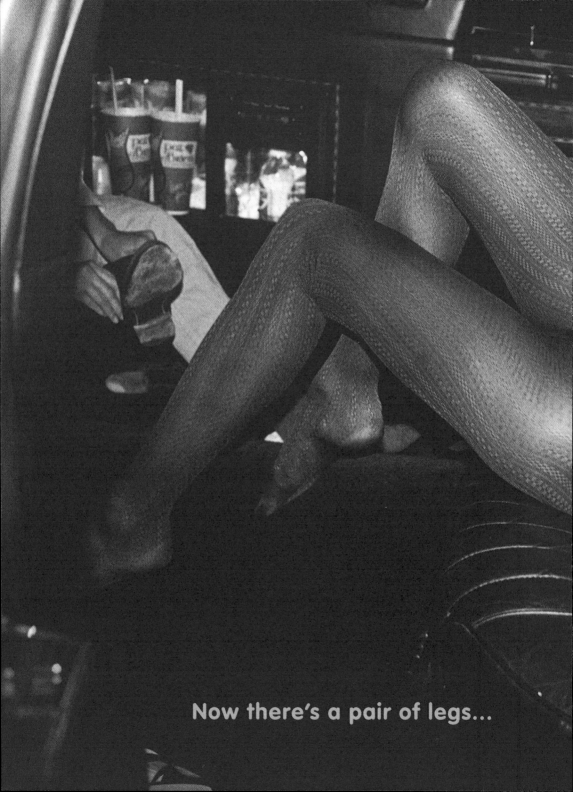

Now there's a pair of legs...

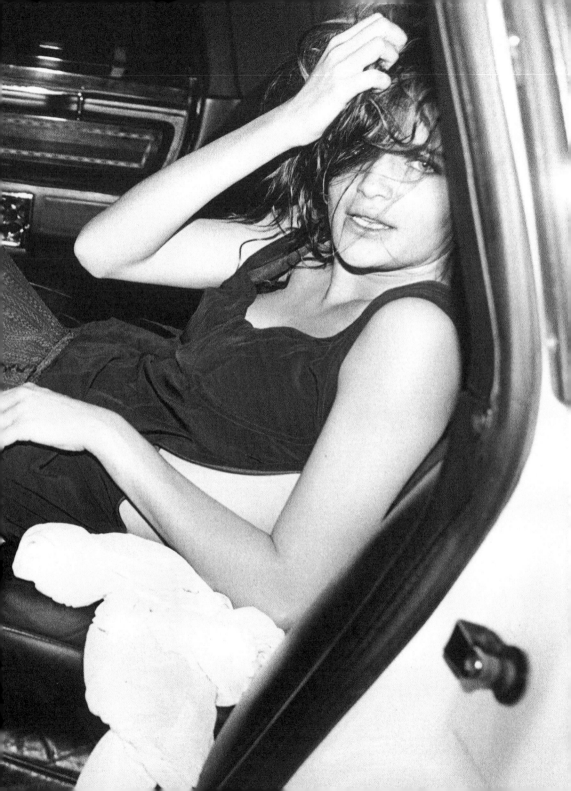

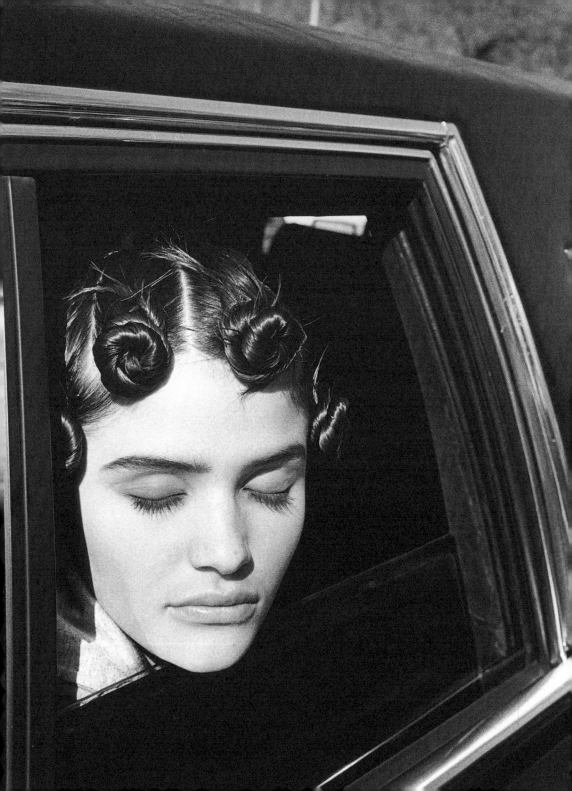

"I love New York because I love junk food."

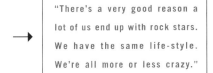

"There's a very good reason a lot of us end up with rock stars. We have the same life-style. We're all more or less crazy."

"I started modeling when I was two years old. By the time I was ten, I hated it. I always wanted to be a writer or an archeologist."

"I like doing the shows. One glass of champagne and my adrenaline gets going."

"I feel my best doing a shoot when I have clothes I feel good in. But what's most important is not what you're wearing but what's on your face. Your eyes always betray your insides."

"How do you get to the top in this business? It helps if you're blonde, have big tits and sleep with all the photographers.... Just kidding."

"MODELING CAN BE BORING WHEN YOU'RE SITTING AROUND IN AIRPORTS ALONE. BUT THAT'S WHAT WE GET PAID FOR, I GUESS."

"I'm perverse—I like dark humor."

"Once I flew for twenty-five hours to Hawaii, was in bed at my hotel at 3 A.M., got up at 5 A.M., was at a shoot all day, got right back on another plane and flew another twenty-five hours back to New York for another shoot. I wake up and think I look like shit, but that's what we have to overcome as models."

"I DON'T MIND BEING PHOTOGRAPHED NUDE. I THINK BARE BREASTS ARE BEAUTIFUL WHETHER THEY'RE LARGE OR SMALL."

tatjana

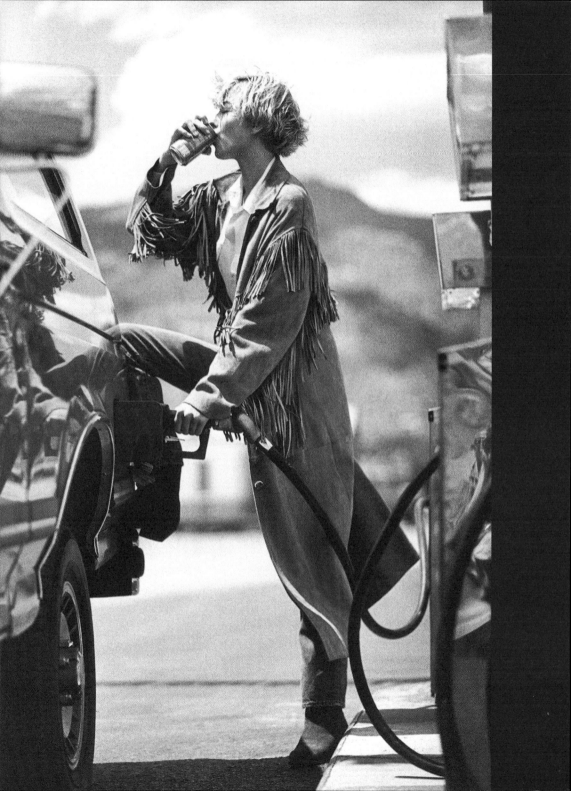

"Why I like modeling: you meet interesting people"

What I wear most: Jeans and a T-shirt. Lately, I like motorcycle boots and Sixties love beads.
What's in my garage: A Bronco. *Why I live where I live:* Now that I'm pursuing an acting career,
I'm in Malibu. Here I can swim, water-ski, keep a zoo—three dogs (a husky, a golden
retriever and a shiatsu), two cats, a cockatoo and a horse.

and make a bundle of money!"

"I'M SO HAPPY I'M GETTING OLDER — I THINK WOMEN LOOK GOOD WITH A LITTLE KNOWLEDGE ON THEIR FACES."

Stephanie's the kind of girl who'd walk into the studio, slap you on the back and help herself to breakfast. She's always up — with a genuine smile and a great sense of humor.

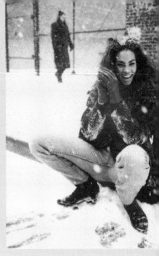

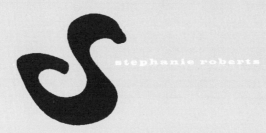

stephanie roberts

"WHEN I FIRST CAME HERE, I STARVED AND PARTIED AND WENT WILD. I HAD NEVER BEEN IN A CITY LIKE NEW YORK BEFORE."

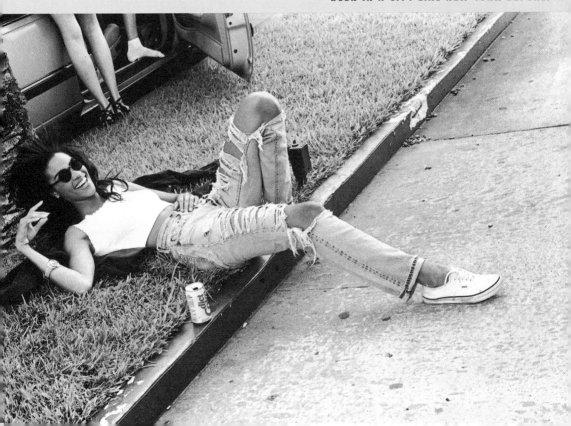

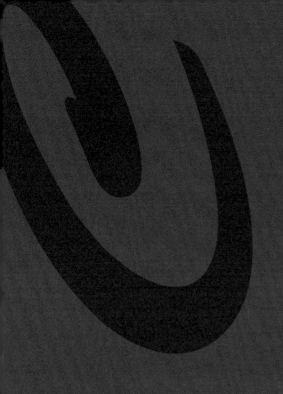

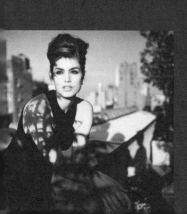

CINDY CRAWFORD

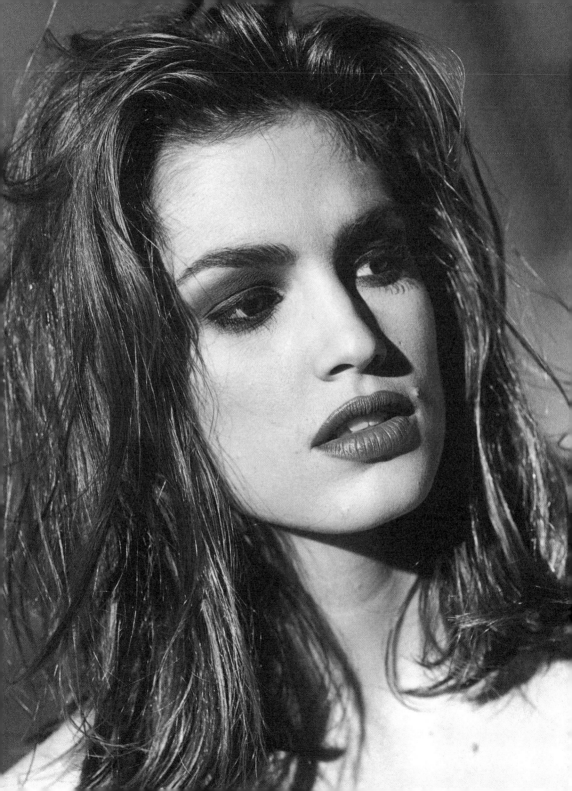

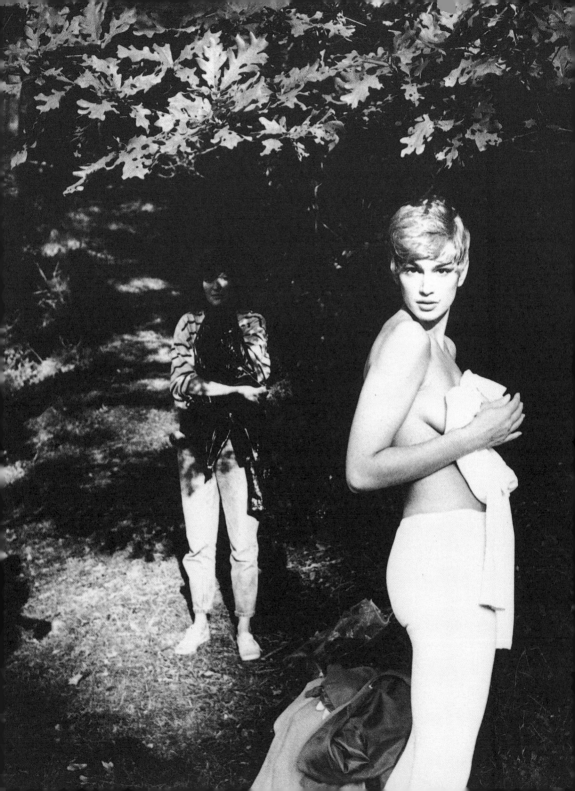

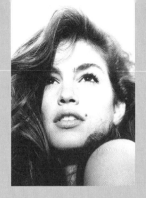

THE FIRST TIME I SAW CINDY

I was shooting for French *Vogue*—I think in 1985. She had a voluptuous, dark glamour that looked very good in a photograph. She had a look that said, "I'm going to do this BIG." It was obvious she was the new generation—that you don't have to be a flat-chested, skinny girl anymore. Cindy has the quintessential cover-girl face. In a photograph, you can see into her eyes—the whites around her eyes. She's really the best for a non-fashion picture—she has that kind of shape that only gets better the more you take away the clothes. She's much more a personality than a clothes hanger. Cindy relates well to crowds when we're shooting on the street. She makes people feel comfortable, posing with them and even interviewing them. I think she will be the next great anchor woman.

CINDY'S PHILOSOPHY

"You have to be a certain height—I don't know why. If you're under five seven, I would say you're not going to make it as a top model. To become a Christy or a Linda, you have to be tall and thin."

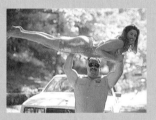

ON THE RUNWAY

"God, I was so scared doing runway the first two years. I hated it. No one teaches you that stuff—you have to figure it out for yourself. I'm just Cindy walking down the runway, and that seems to be all right for now. It's hard sometimes because I feel silly."

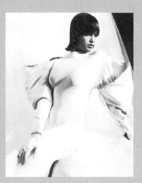

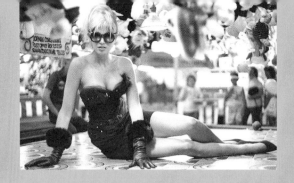

"I like clothes, but that doesn't mean I want to spend half an hour every morning figuring out what I'm going to wear. Absolutely not."

"I'M SO LUCKY. Modeling has invited me to see the world. Here I was, this girl from DeKalb, Illinois, living in New York this life-style that people think is so glamorous. It is sometimes. I mean, even stupid things like food. I didn't know what smoked salmon or fresh mozzarella was until I came here. Modeling has introduced me to all these flavors of life.

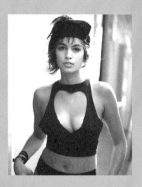

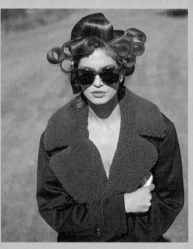

"I grew up eating Cheez Whiz and Wonder Bread, so I've had to educate myself about eating properly. I don't eat meat, and I stay away from dairy products. I've learned to cook, and I eat out at restaurants that serve healthy food."

"When I'm working with good photographers who I feel a rapport with, I don't think about anything but the picture. On more boring jobs, I like to think about my grocery list or decorating my apartment. I'd rather my mind be on the photograph, but there aren't that many jobs that inspire me anymore."

She is a model *with* a mission

"My father always says, 'They don't call this work for nothing.' It's a great job most of the time. But there are some days when you just have to keep your chin up. Basically, the thing about modeling is that if you're smart and you can save money when you're thirty, you can do whatever you want. It's such a luxury to decide what you want to do."

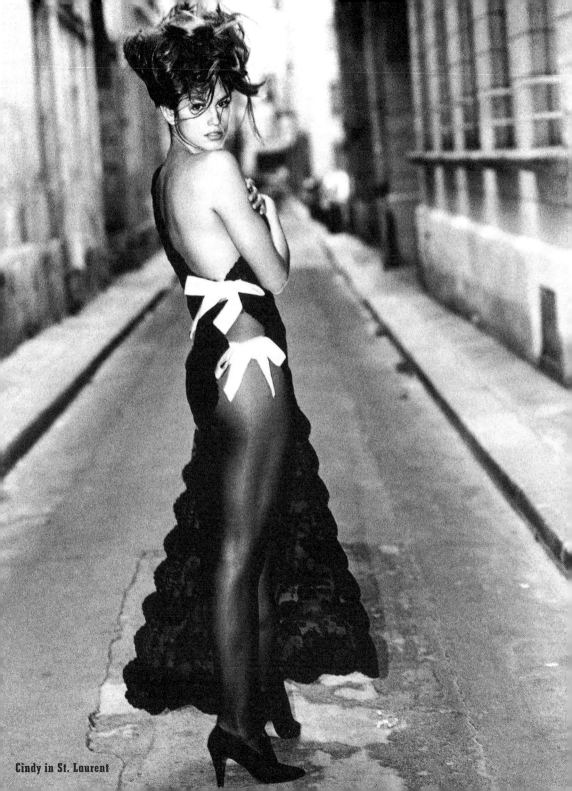

Cindy in St. Laurent

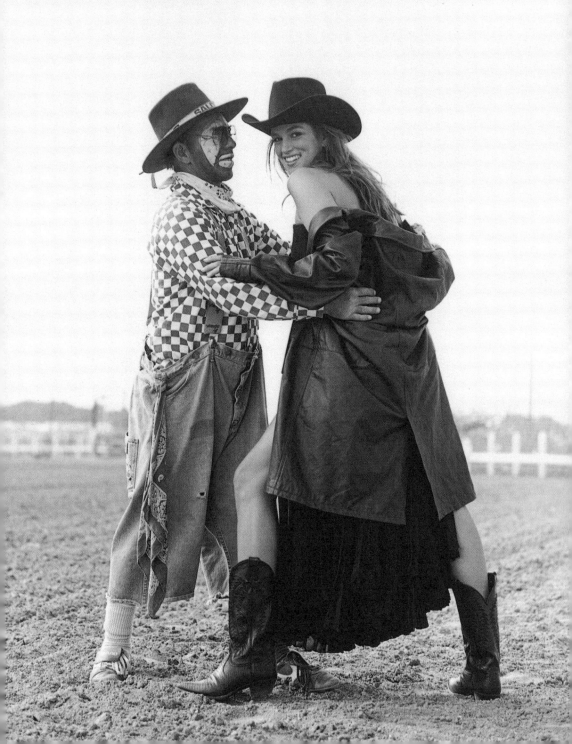

"It's a full-time job keeping yourself together. When I'm not working, if I take a week off, I'm never bored because I'm getting bikini and leg waxings, pedicures, facials and working out with my trainer."

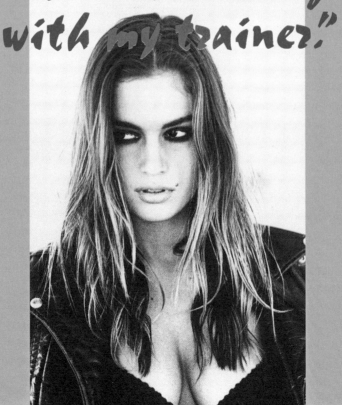

THIS IS WYOMING. I ASKED CHARLENE IF SHE

WOULD BE OUT ON THIS ROAD AT 6:30 A.M.,

WHEN THE LIGHT WAS GOOD. SOMETIMES

THERE ARE SACRIFICES TO BE MADE.

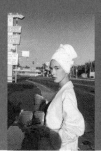

SUSAN HOLMES, READY TO GO

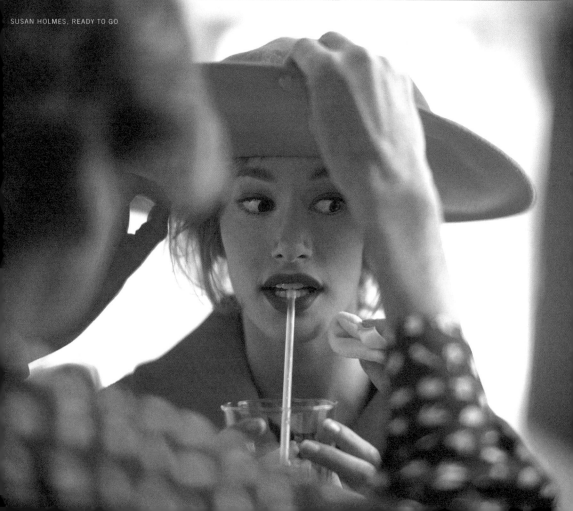

AND HANGING AROUND

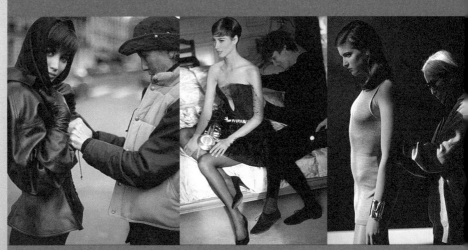

CHRISTY TURLINGTON AND POLLY MELLEN IN PARIS.   CHRISTY GETS PINNED BY GRACE CODDINGTON.   POLLY PREPS STEPHANIE SEYMOUR.

One of the realities of this job is that everyone has to show up before the shoot—the makeup artist, the hairdresser, the fashion editor. It's their role to glorify the model. It's the one real thing that we do. The rest is fantasy.

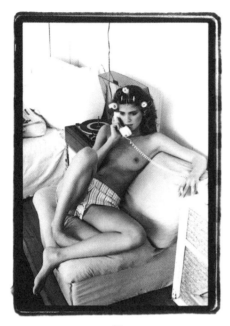

GIA

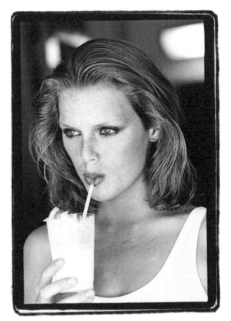

PATTI HANSEN

GETTING READY FOR A SHOOT IS THE PRELUDE IN OUR PROFESSION. UNLIKE THE JOB, WE'RE NOT HAVING TO MAKE ANYTHING HAPPEN. IT'S LIKE BEING BACK-STAGE AT THE THEATER, WHERE I'M A PRIVILEGED OBSERVER. SINCE HAIR AND MAKEUP CAN TAKE ANYWHERE FROM ONE AND A HALF TO TWO HOURS, THIS IS THE BEST TIME FOR ME TO WARM UP, TO GET TO KNOW WHO I'M GOING TO PHOTOGRAPH, TO SNAP SOME PICTURES WHILE THE GIRL IS AT HER MOST RELAXED. I GET TO BE RELAXED AND GET IN THE MOOD, TOO. ONE OF MY FAVORITE PHOTOS IS OF PATTI HANSEN DRINKING A PIÑA COLADA FROM A STRAW WHILE SHE'S HAVING HER HAIR DONE. SHE WASN'T READY. THE HAIRDRESSER SAID, "SHE'S NOT READY." I SAID, "OF COURSE SHE'S READY" AND SHOT THE PICTURE. MOST MODELS DON'T MIND THE INTRUSION. I'VE ALWAYS BEEN A RATHER VOYEURISTIC SNAPPER, SO THE FACT THAT I'VE ALWAYS DONE IT AND BEEN OBVIOUS ABOUT IT ALMOST MAKES IT SEEM NAT-URAL. SOME OF MY OTHER FAVORITES ARE OF GIA IN ROLLERS LYING ON A BED TALK-ING ON THE PHONE, JERRY HALL HAVING A CIGARETTE AND SUSAN HESS POSING WHILE SOMEBODY WAS TAKING LIGHT READINGS. I IMMEDIATELY RELATE TO THESE PICTURES—FOR ME, THEY COME CLOSEST TO THE TRUTH OF IT ALL.

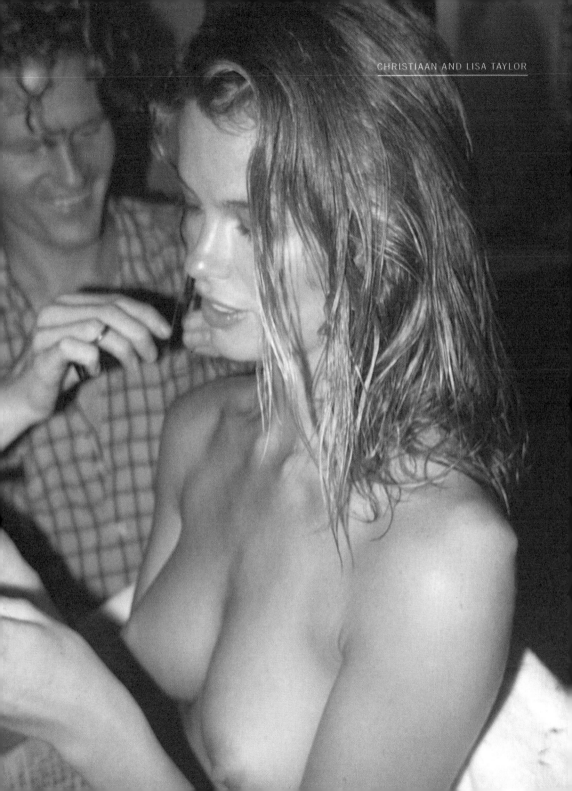

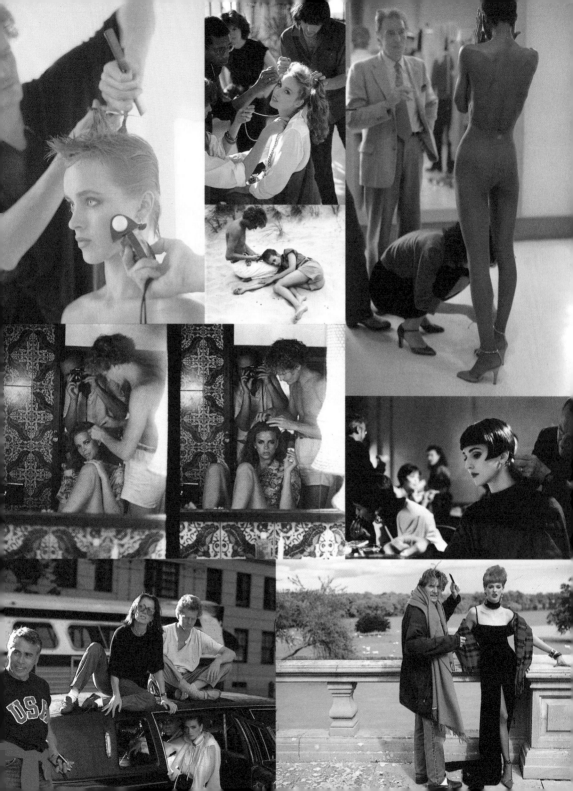

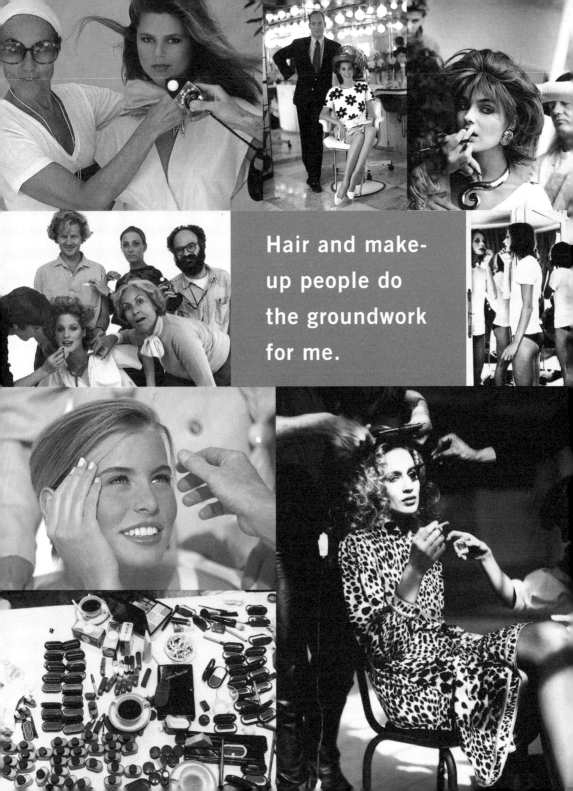

Hair and make-up people do the groundwork for me.

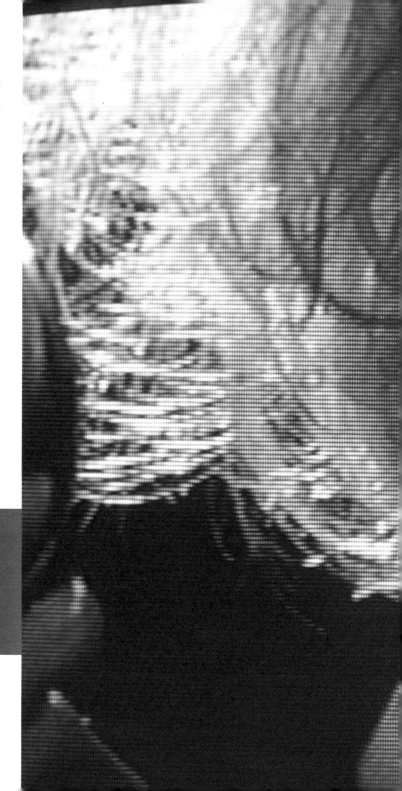

THE MAKEUP, THE HAIR ARE RITUALISTIC ACTS THAT BRING EVERYONE CLOSE TO ONE ANOTHER. WONDERFUL THINGS HAPPEN IN THE PREPARATION. AT THIS TIME, YOU'RE PART OF SOMETHING REAL. I ALWAYS LIKE "BEFORE" SHOTS—A MODEL USUALLY LOOKS VERY GOOD WHEN SOMEONE'S TOUCHING HER. IT'S LIKE A MASSAGE. THE HAIRDRESSER AND MAKEUP ARTISTS LEARN EVERYTHING ABOUT A GIRL BECAUSE THERE'S AN ELECTRICITY BETWEEN THEM. ONE OF THE THINGS I SAY TO MODELS, A RULE, IS THAT

JENY HOWORTH: "I always loved having my makeup done. But even after ten years, I still can't get a straight pencil line around my lips."

IF YOU CAN LOOK AS GOOD AS YOU DO NOW ALL DAY, IT WILL BE PERFECT.

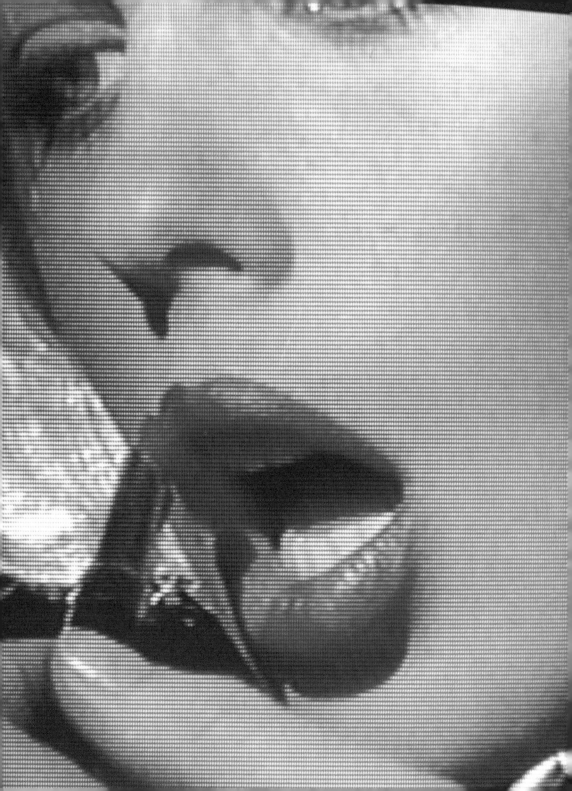

hair and makeup

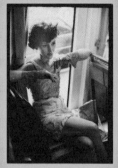

WENDY WHITELAW

I like the way a model looks when she first walks in the door, so my favorite hair and makeup artists are the ones who can make the girls look as though they're not made-up at all. The people I like to work with go beyond doing hair and makeup. They get involved in the shoot and contribute to the story on other levels.

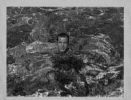

VINCENT NASSO

VALENTIN

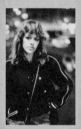

ARIELLA

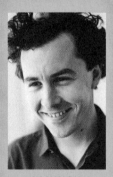

YANNICK

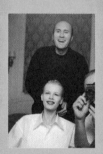

SERGE NORMANT

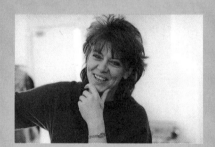

HEIDI MORAWETZ

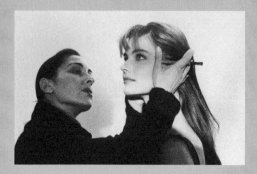

LYDIA SCHNEIDER

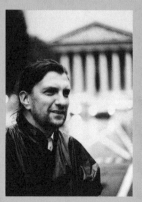

DIDIER MALIGE

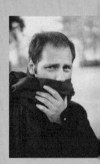

BOBBY BOOTS

They not only get the girl ready, they make friends with the girl, get her relaxed. Meanwhile, I'm warming up while all this is happening, moving around, quietly snapping away. It's easier to be with the model at this time. It's not, Okay, and now give me my camera.

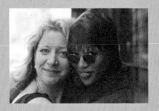

MARY GREENWELL AND NAOMI

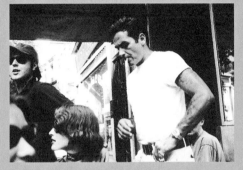

FRANCOIS NARS   ORIBE

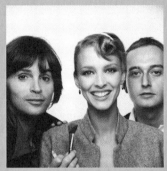

WAY BANDY, KAREN BJORNSON, ROBERT TURNER

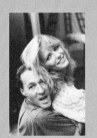

MAURY HOBSON AND
CHERYL TIEGS

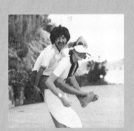

SUGA AND YASMIN

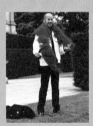

LAURIE

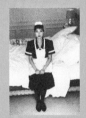

BRIGITTE REISS
ANDERSEN

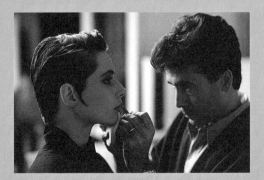

ISABELLA ROSSELLINI AND THIBAUD

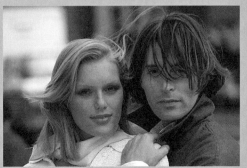

PATTI HANSEN AND
WAY BANDY

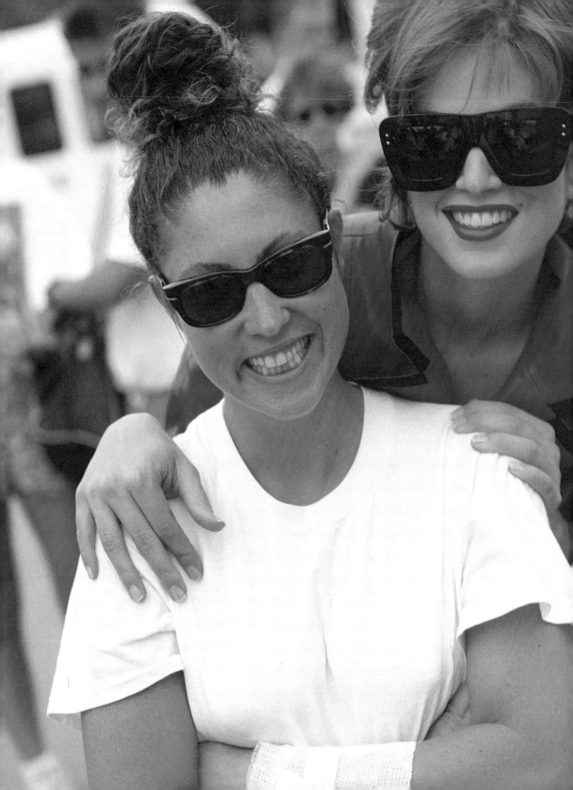

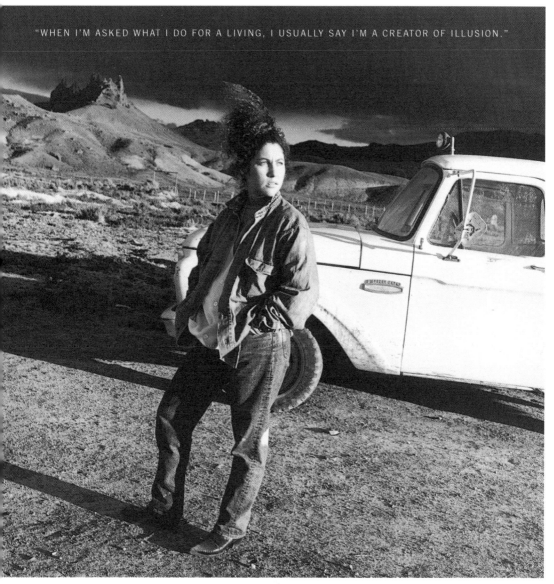

"WHEN I'M ASKED WHAT I DO FOR A LIVING, I USUALLY SAY I'M A CREATOR OF ILLUSION."

SONIA KASHUK

"It really does come down to everybody working together and trying to make the girl feel beautiful. My role is to make her feel the most comfortable she can be. Because if she's not, the picture is not going to work. I don't like transforming girls into something else. Makeup should be an enhancer, not a transformer. Sometimes my job is all about understanding what *not* to do. If we're on the beach, I might get paid to say a model doesn't need anything on her face. It's all about maintaining the quality of the girl. If you leave the skin real, she stays real."

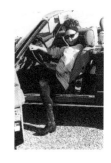

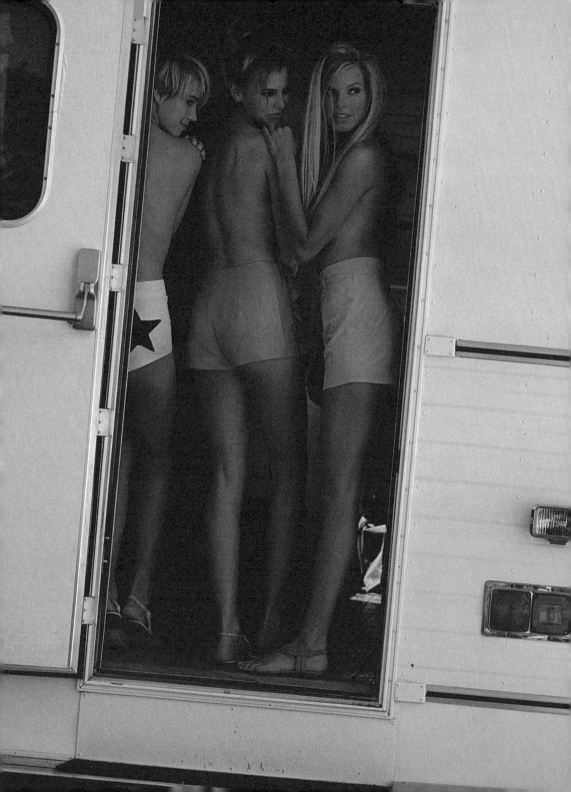

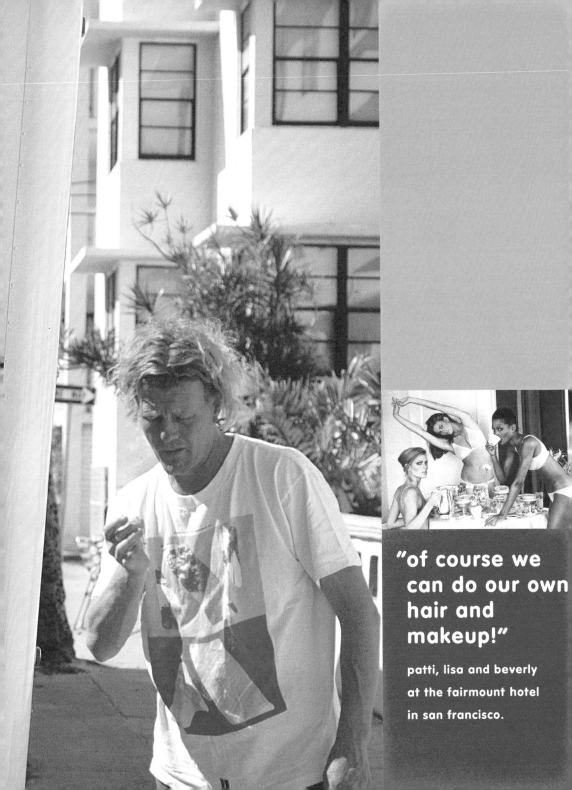

"of course we can do our own hair and makeup!"

patti, lisa and beverly at the fairmount hotel in san francisco.

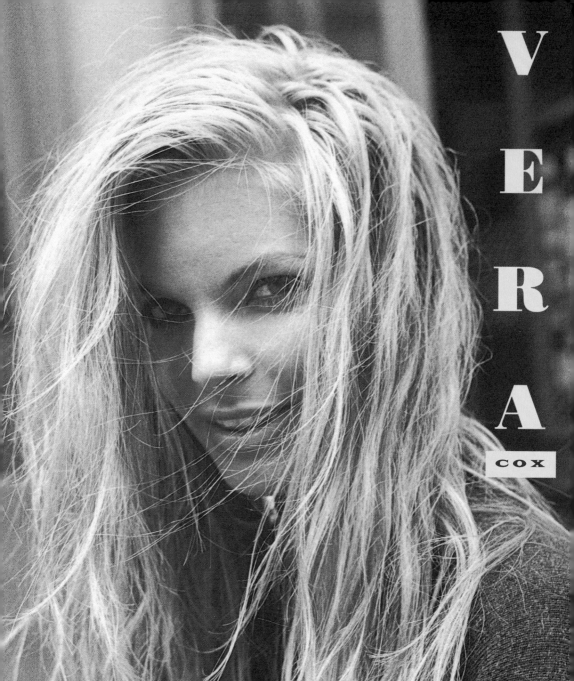

V
E
R
A

COX

"WHAT YOU DO AS A MODEL IN FRONT OF THE CAMERA IS NOT A LEARNED THING—YOU EITHER HAVE IT OR YOU DON'T."

WHEN I FIRST SAW HER, SHE WAS VERY DANDY AND HAD HER COWBOY BOOTS ON . . . .
SHE'S WISE AND PROVOCATIVE.

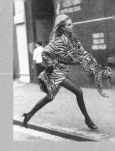

Q: Do you ever wake up in the morning and think you look like hell? A: All the time!

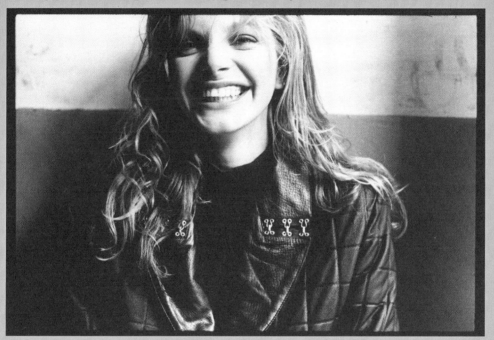

"Modeling is great. But it can be damaging, because you're depending
on your looks. I'm lucky—I always feel beautiful from the inside.
I'm my own little cheerleader, thanks to my family."

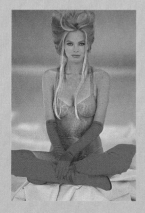

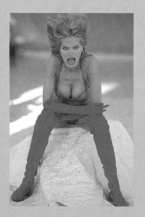

"THERE IS NO LOGIC IN
THIS BUSINESS. IT CAN BE
FRUSTRATING—EVEN IF
YOU DO YOUR HOMEWORK
AND WORK HARD, THERE
ARE NO GUARANTEES. YOU
CAN HAVE A PERFECT CHIN,
PERFECT HAIR, A GREAT
SMILE—YOU CAN HAVE IT
ALL AND NOT DO WELL.
THERE'S NO FORMULA."

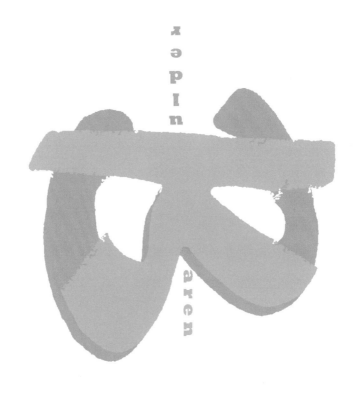

"I'M VERY NORMAL."

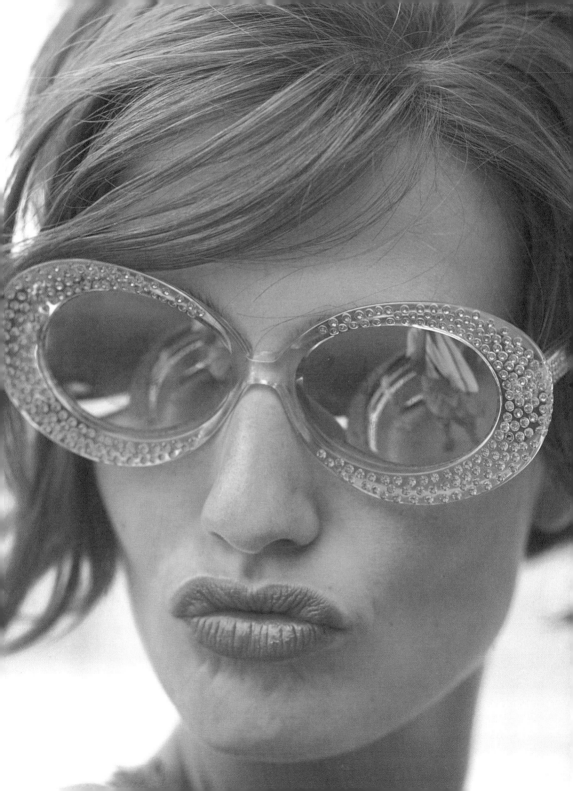

THE WORLD ALWAYS NEEDS A NEW BLONDE

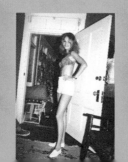

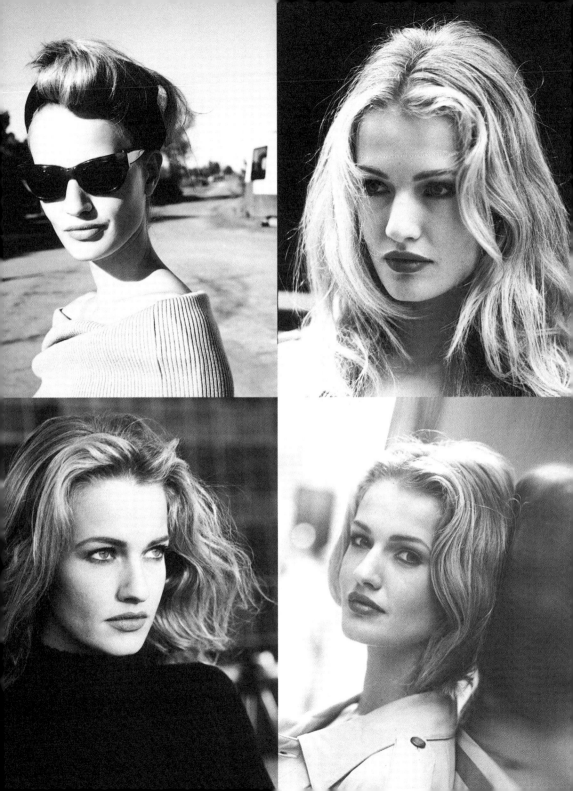

"WHEN I WAS YOUNG, I THOUGHT I WAS UGLY. I'M FIVE FOOT TEN, AND BACK THEN I FELT HUGE AND AWKWARD. BUT SOMETIMES IT'S A PLUS TO BE INSECURE. IT MAKES YOU TRY HARDER. ● **WHAT COULD BE BETTER THAN TO BE YOUNG AND BEAUTIFUL AND MAKE A LOT OF MONEY?"** ●

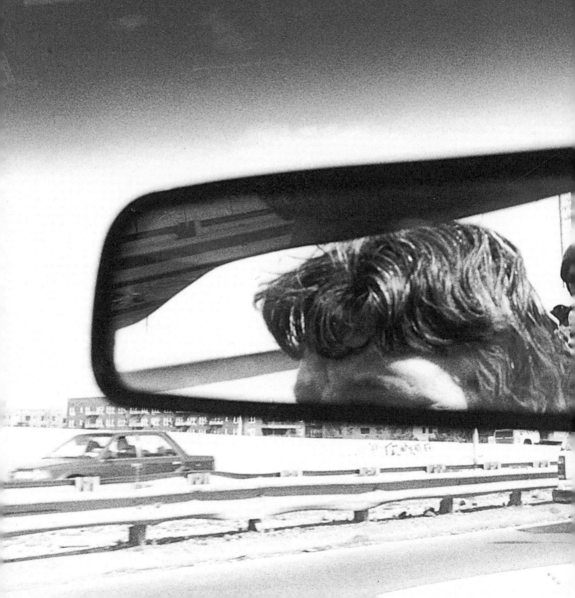

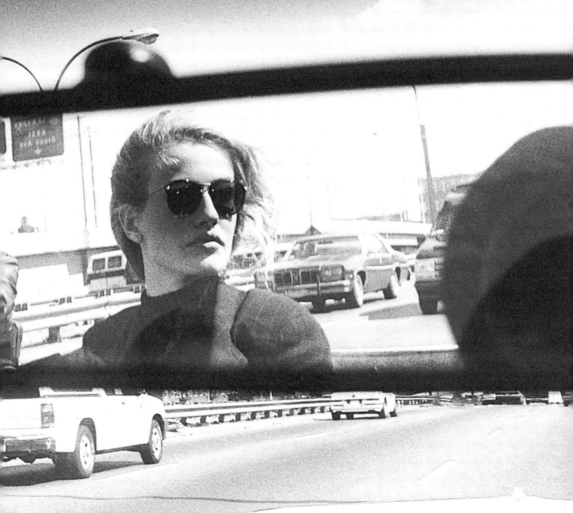

"WHEN I FIRST STARTED MODELING, I STILL HAD BRACES ON MY TEETH. ● THE FIRST TIME I HAD MY PICTURE TAKEN, THEY WERE SHOOTING LINGERIE. THEY SENT ME HOME BECAUSE I LOOKED SO SCARED." ●

"PEOPLE THINK MODELS ARE STUPID. OF COURSE THEY'RE NOT. THEY'RE JUST NOT ADULTS YET."

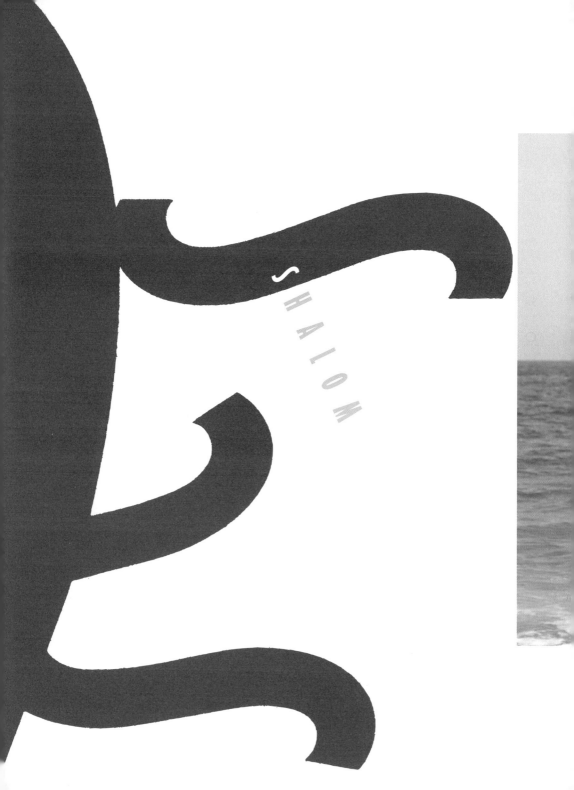

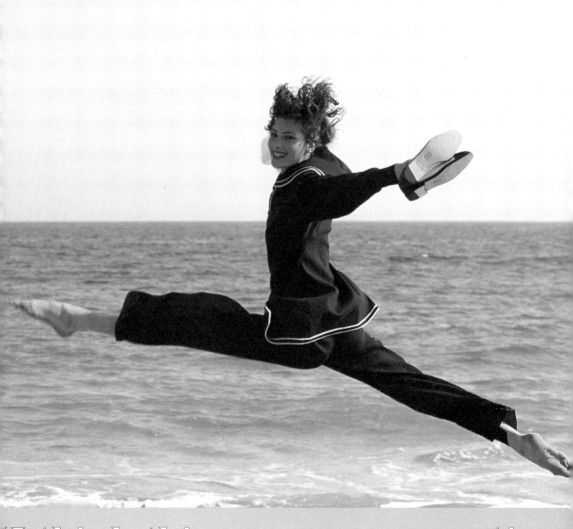

'I think this younger generation of models is a lot less concerned with stardom. And I think that's a nice change."

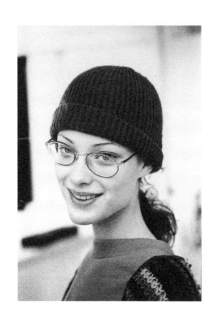
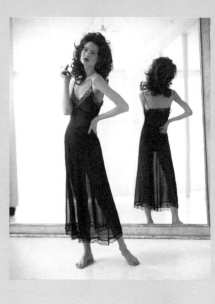
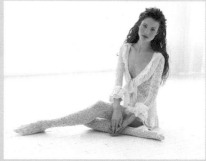
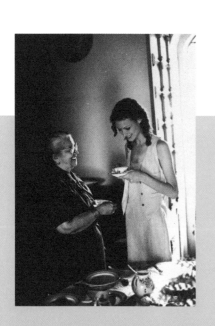
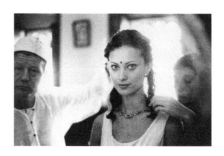

How are you today?

I'm peachy keen.

How did you get your name?

"Shalom" means "Peace be with you" in Hebrew.

What is your family like?

My parents were hippies. I was a vegetarian until I was eight. My mum made all our clothes and baked bread. My dad was a social worker. Now he dabbles in real estate.

Why do you think that suddenly everyone wants to work with you?

I suppose it has to do with looks—height and bone structure and all. But I'm also a really open person, and I'm not afraid to do anything.

What does it take to be a model?

When I first started, I thought you had to be all, you know, "Do model pose number one." But watching other girls helps. And taking direction from the photographer.

What model do you most admire?

Linda Evangelista. She pulls out everything and looks completely relaxed and natural.

What do you do if you hate the clothes you have to wear?

I just think of how to improve them rather than bitch about it. If I'm jumping, the clothes look better.

What do you like to eat?

When I'm home with my parents, it's vegetables and rice cakes. In New York, I eat pizza and ice cream.

Do you exercise?

Not much. I live on the sixth floor of a building and I run up and down those stairs at least ten times a day.

How much sleep do you need?

Well, I'm young, so I can get away with having three hours and still look pretty good in the morning.

Do you drink or do drugs?

I don't drink much. I've been smoking pot since I was fourteen, but never on the job.

Where do you shop?

Flea markets and thrift shops.

Who's your favorite actress?

Lauren Bacall because she's classy.

What can't you live without in your life?

My best friends Amber, John and Sam.

Is modeling easy?

No. You work your ass off for four months, every day plus Saturdays and Sundays, and then all of a sudden you're free for a month and a half.

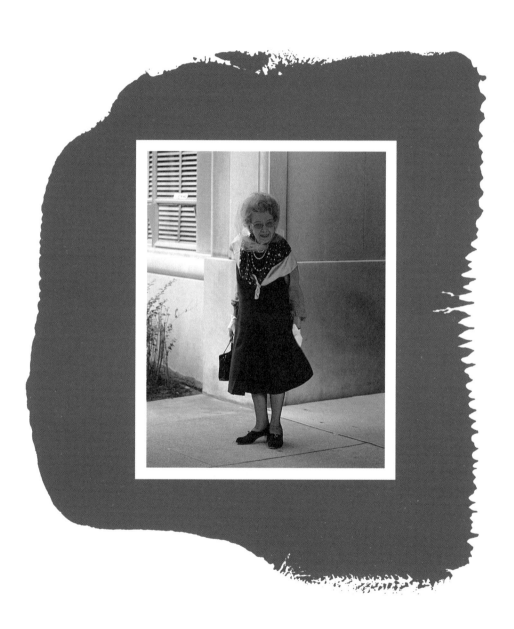

living

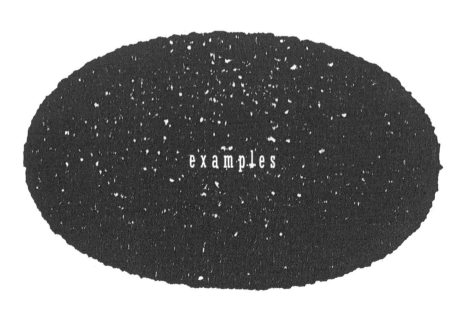

examples

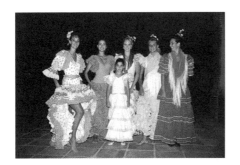

WHEN I'M ON LOCATION, I LIKE TO LOOK AROUND ME BEFORE

SHOOTING ANY PICTURES. THIS GIVES ME AN OPPORTUNITY TO

OBSERVE REAL PEOPLE IN REAL SITUATIONS. I MIGHT SEE AN OLD

LADY PAUSING IN A DOORWAY OR A GROUP OF YOUNG GIRLS

STANDING AROUND LAUGHING AND TALKING ANIMATEDLY. THESE

ARE WHAT I CALL LIVING EXAMPLES—THEY GIVE ME AND THE

MODEL A GOOD STARTING POINT FOR TELLING A FASHION STORY.

I CAN SAY TO HER, "I DON'T WANT YOU TO MODEL, I JUST WANT

YOU TO DO WHAT YOU SEE THAT WOMAN OVER THERE DOING."

WHEN THE MODEL HAS TO CONCENTRATE ON BEING IN A SITUA-

TION INSTEAD OF WHERE SHE'S PUTTING HER FEET AND HANDS,

SHE CAN LET HERSELF GO AND LOOK MUCH MORE RELAXED.

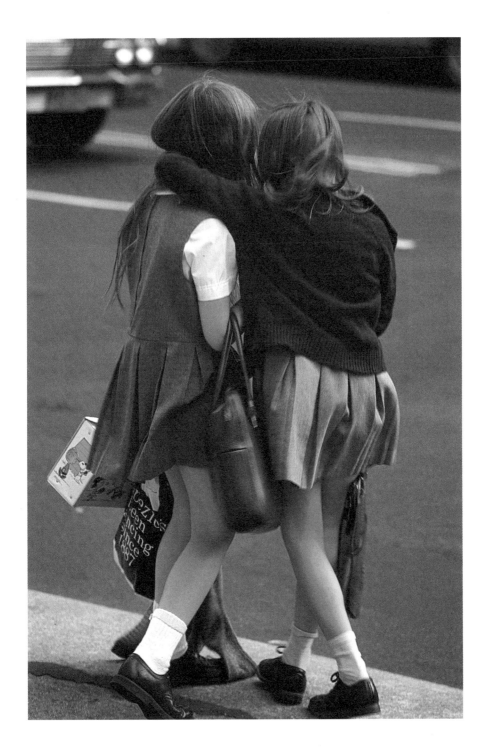

When I see schoolgirls together, I like to remind the model that she needs to keep that sense of innocence and charm—that she can still be a child.

YOU SEE THE
WAY THAT
GENTLEMAN
IS WALKING
ACROSS THE
STREET,
HOLDING THAT
NEWSPAPER?

NOW YOU
DO THAT.

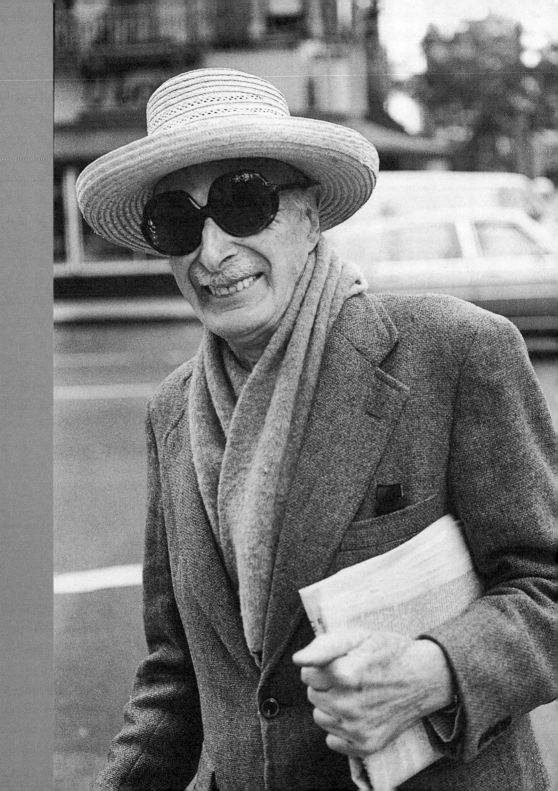

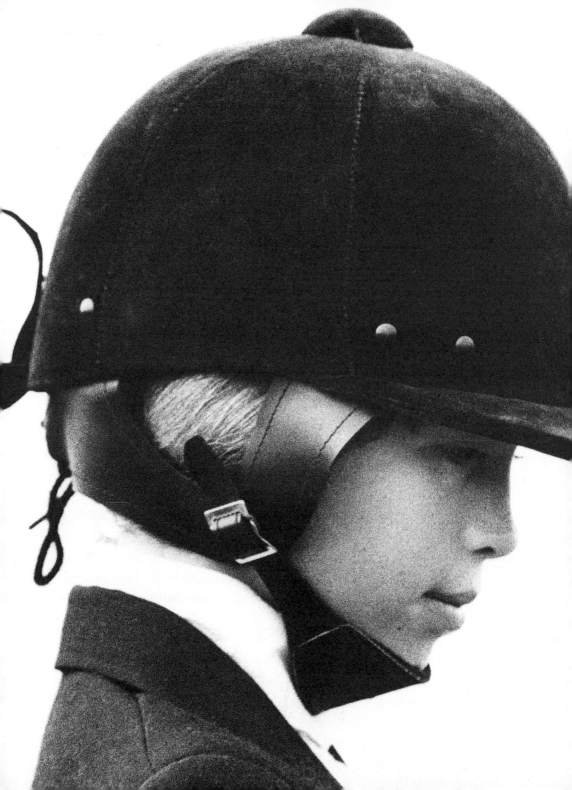

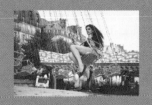

It doesn't matter whether a girl is wearing riding breeches or a Chanel suit. A uniform makes taking the picture that much easier.

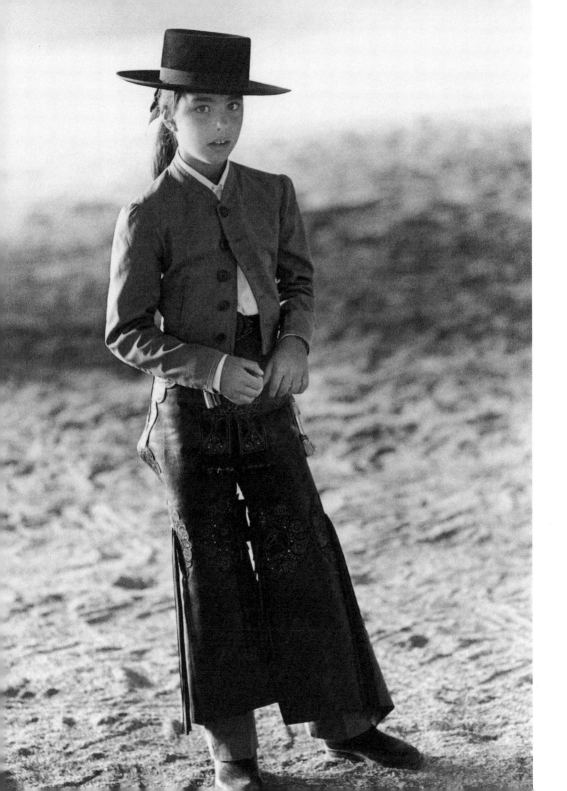

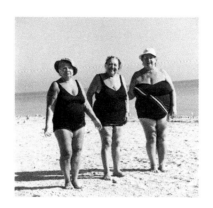

You don't have to act like a model. Learn to relax, like these ladies.

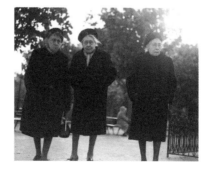

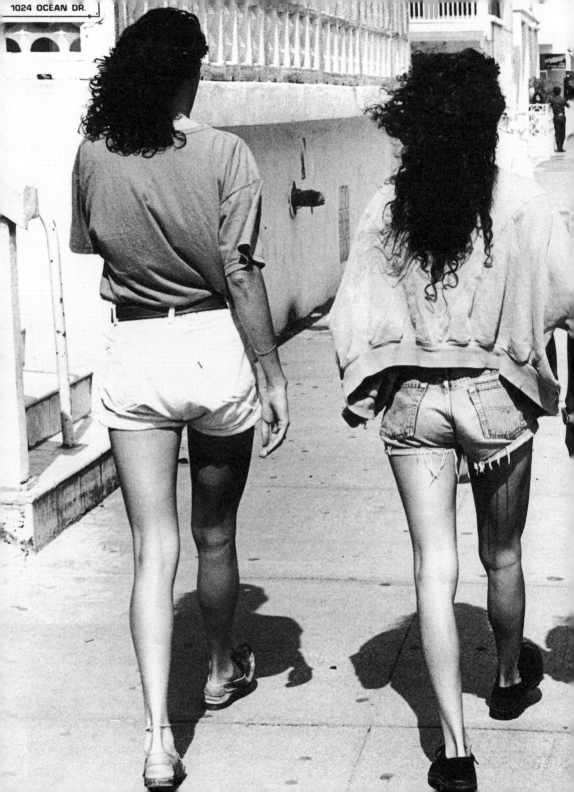

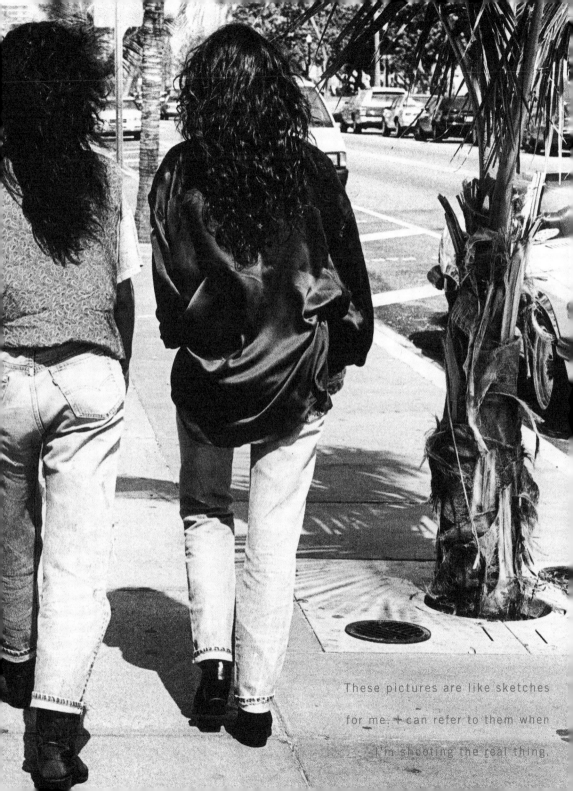

These pictures are like sketches for me. I can refer to them when I'm shooting the real thing.

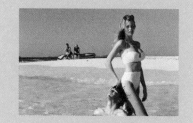

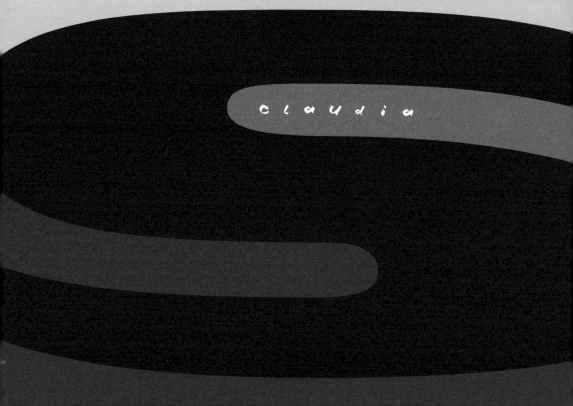

claudia

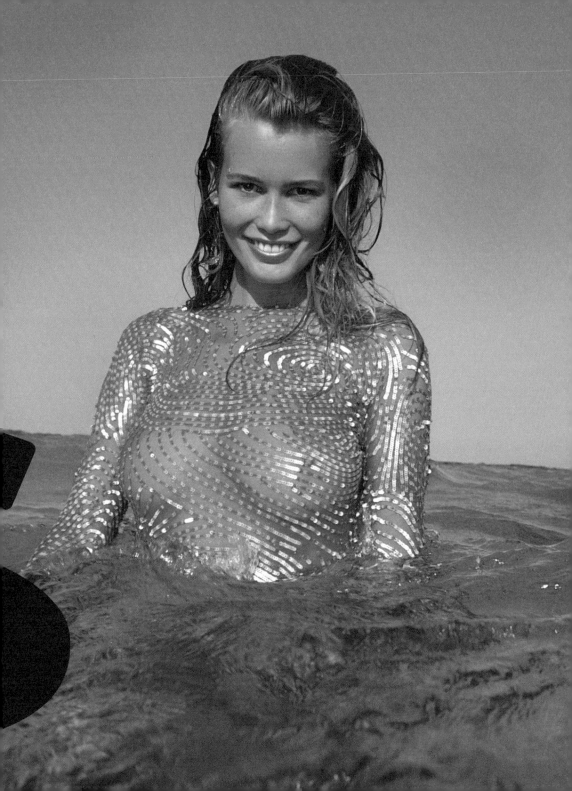

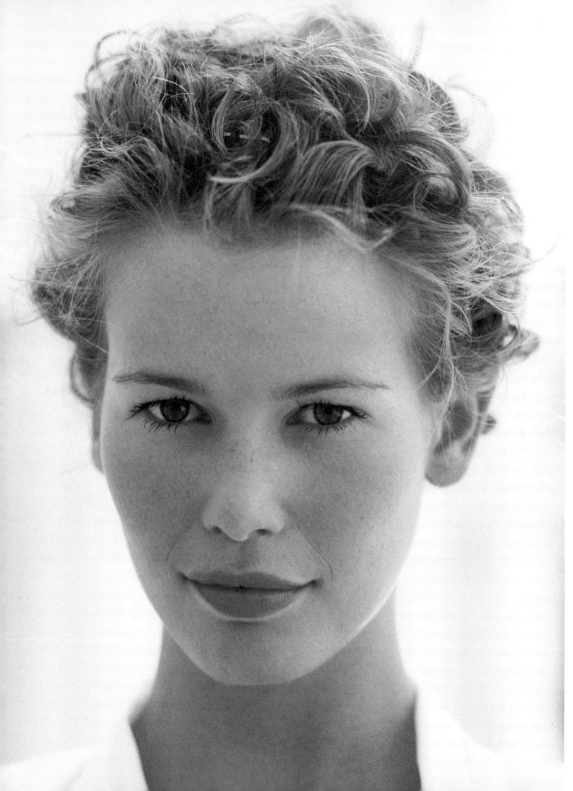

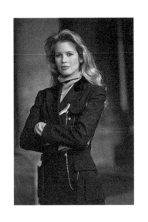

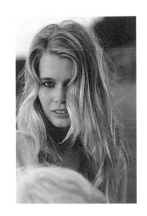

She's more like a movie star than a model. Strangers will approach Claudia on the street for autographs—once, on location, I couldn't believe the crowds at our table while we were eating. She just smiles and sighs.

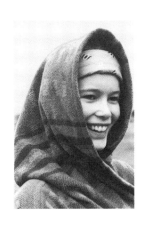

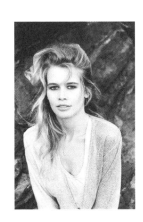

"Claudia is the proto-type of the woman a man dreams about— blonde, with that face. Very Brigitte Bardot.

—Carlyne Cerf de Dudzeele

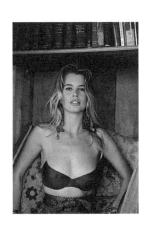

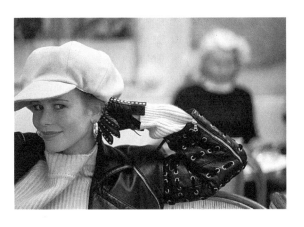

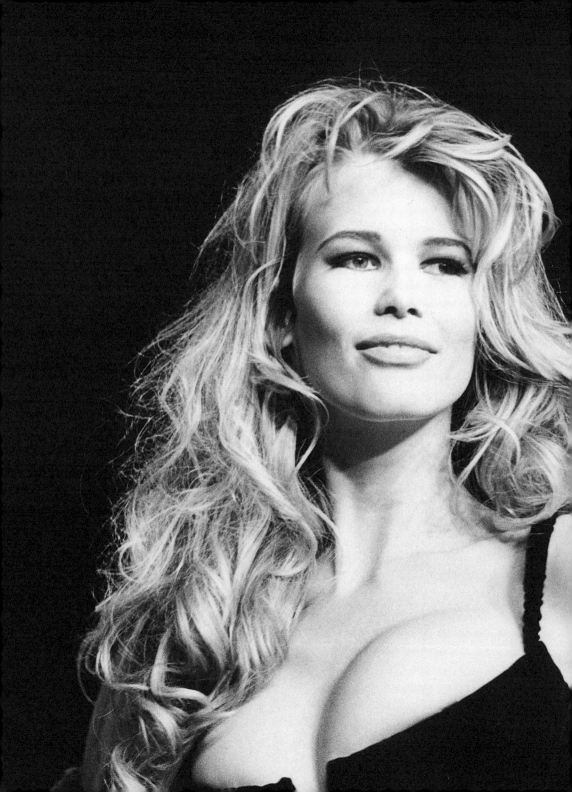

claudia schiffer
is bigger than life

N U D

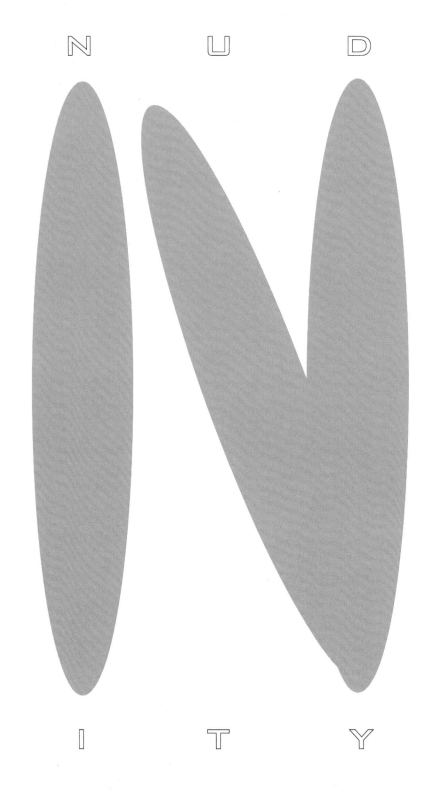

I T Y

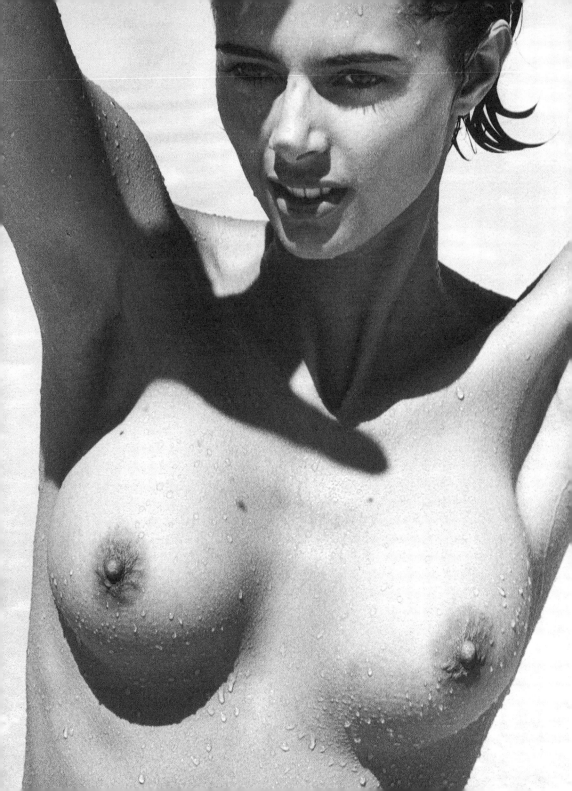

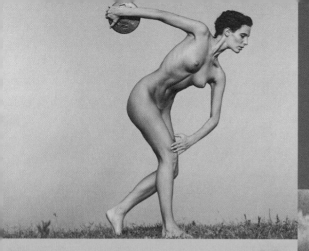

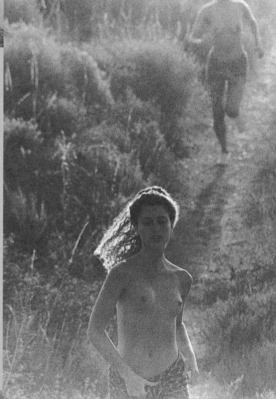

HELENA CHRISTENSEN:

"I DON'T MIND BEING PHOTOGRAPHED NUDE. I THINK BARE BREASTS ARE BEAUTIFUL."

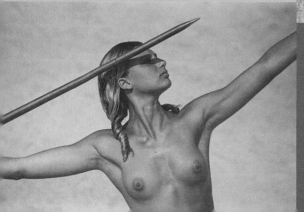

The opportunity to shoot someone in the nude usually comes at off-hours—before a shoot, before the hair and makeup and fiddling. Or when the day is done and everyone wants to relax. If you're on location, it might happen around a pool. It's the one part of the day that feels real.

It's not about big or small breasts. If a model is skinny and flat-chested but has good posture, shooting nude can be great. It's really only if she's wearing clothes that the right body matters. Then she'd better be long legged.

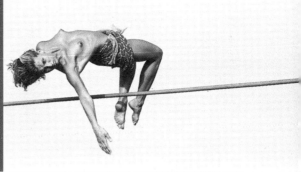

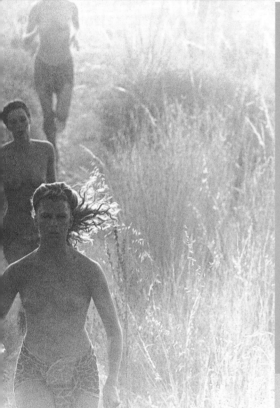

THE PLEASURE OF NUDITY IS THAT IT'S TIMELESS. IT'S WHY I LIKE PONYTAILS AND WET HAIR—WHENEVER A HAIRDO OR OUTFIT ENTERS INTO THE PICTURE, YOU'RE PUTTING A DATE ON THE PHOTO. I WANT TO BE ABLE TO LOOK AT MY PICTURES AND THINK THAT I JUST TOOK THEM. THE ENGLISH GIRLS ARE THE LEAST SELF-CONSCIOUS AND THE MOST COMFORTABLE WITH THEIR BODIES—LIKE HEATHER WHYTE. WHEN THE MODEL IS AT EASE, AS THE PHOTOGRAPHER, YOU NEVER FEEL YOU'RE PART OF SOME TRICK TO TRY TO GET HER TO TAKE HER CLOTHES OFF. THAT'S NOT WHAT IT'S ALL ABOUT.

Paulina: "I was part of the Christie Brinkley era—we had that all-American look. Nudity was shocking. But I'm typically European, so for me, it was no problem."

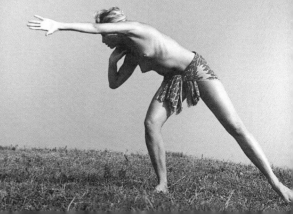

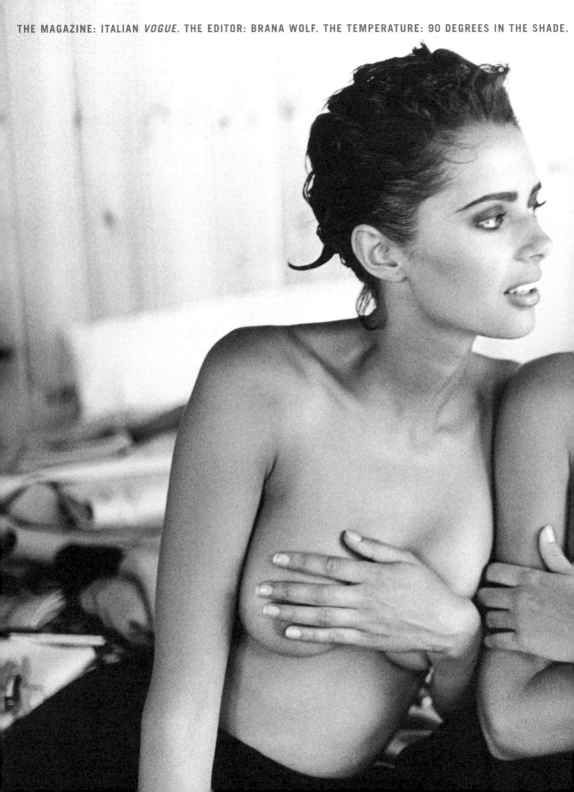

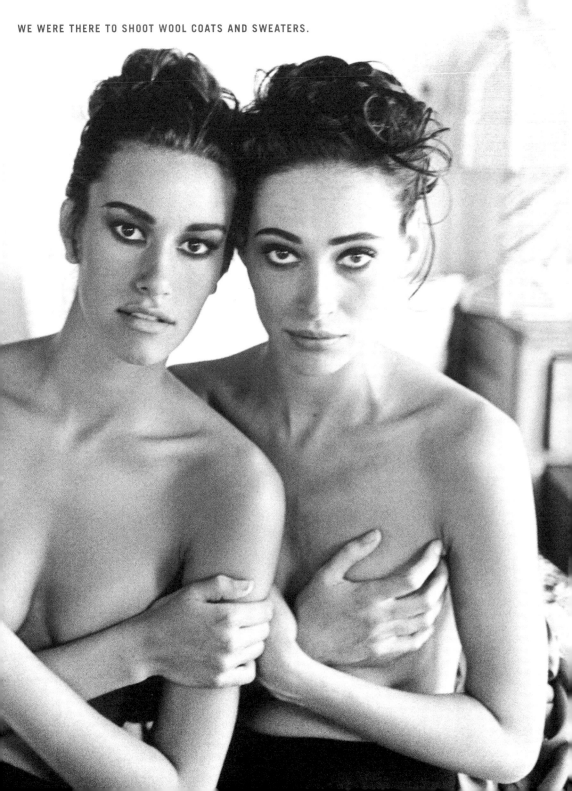

A great model is *comfortable*

in her body without clothes

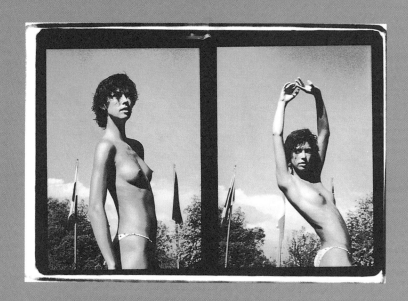

and that makes me...

Comfortable

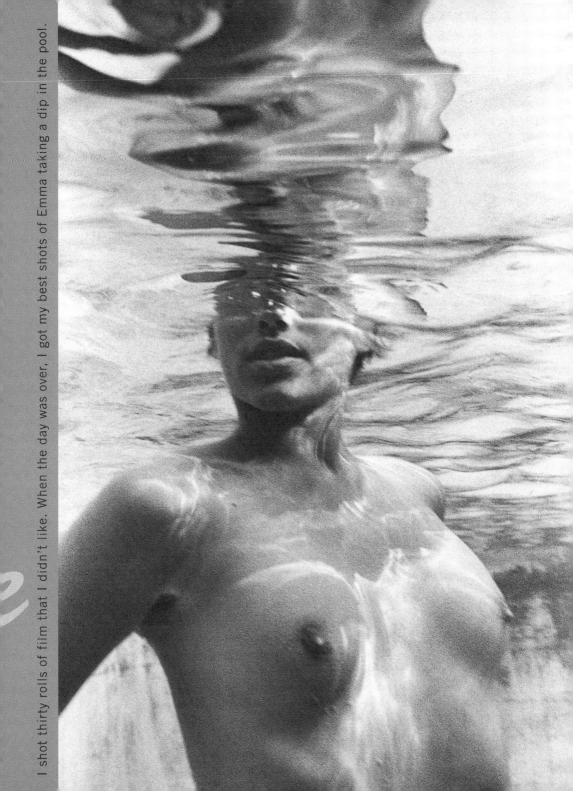

I shot thirty rolls of film that I didn't like. When the day was over, I got my best shots of Emma taking a dip in the pool.

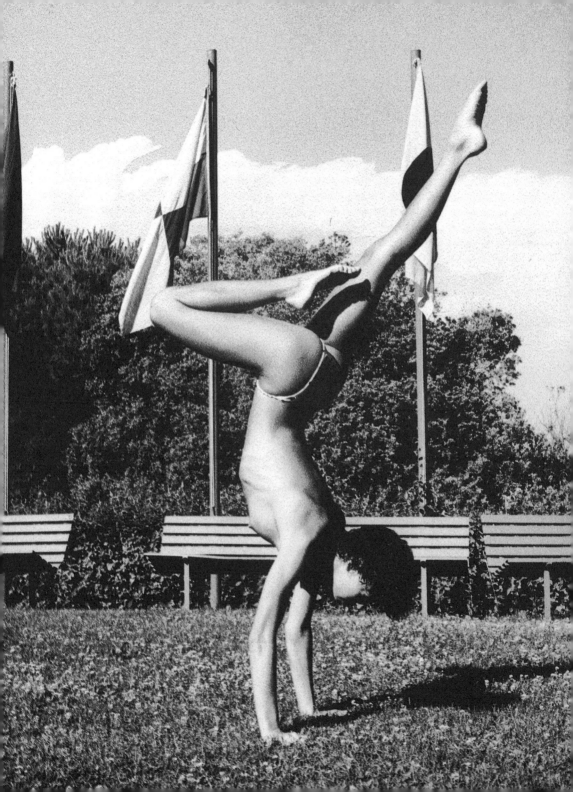

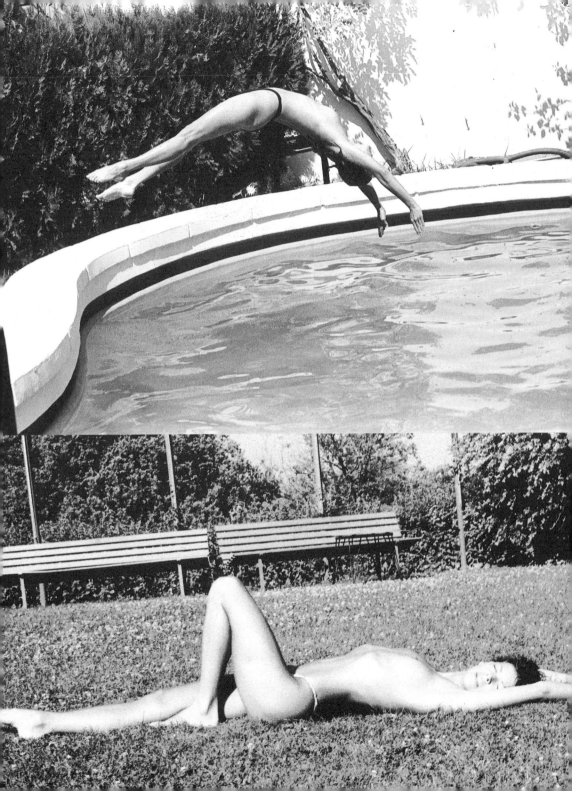

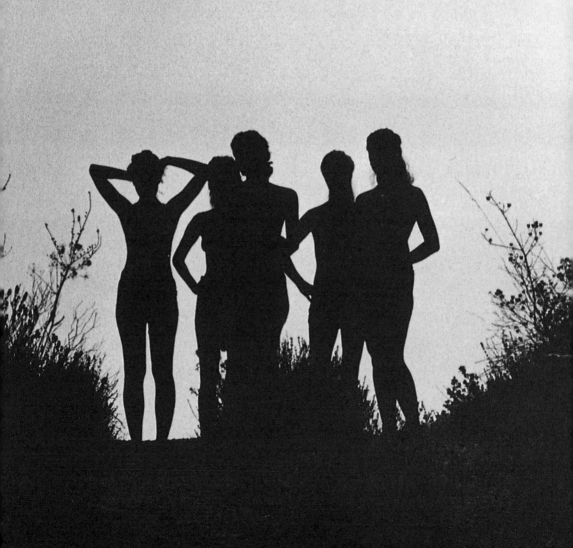

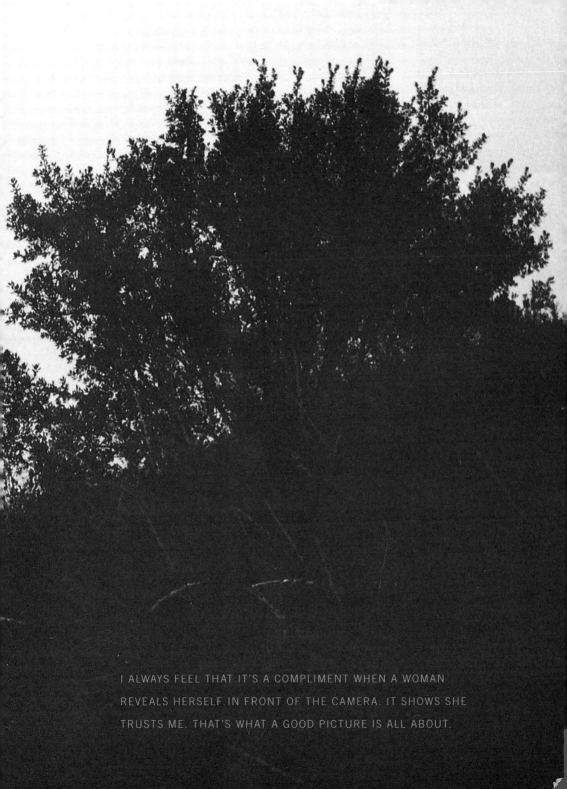

I ALWAYS FEEL THAT IT'S A COMPLIMENT WHEN A WOMAN
REVEALS HERSELF IN FRONT OF THE CAMERA. IT SHOWS SHE
TRUSTS ME. THAT'S WHAT A GOOD PICTURE IS ALL ABOUT.

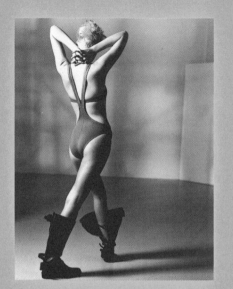

"**I**t all started when I was seventeen years old and had green hair. I was going to the hairdresser to get it changed to pink or something like that. The salon on Baker Street in London was below the Select modeling agency. Someone from the agency told me that I should be a model. I thought it was all kind of seedy and horrible, so I sent my dad to talk to them to make sure it was all aboveboard. ■ The agency told me I couldn't model with pink hair, so I changed it to orange. The only person who would hire me was Michael Roberts. We did the *London Sunday Times*, and then I went to Paris for *Marie Claire.* ■ When I shaved my hair off and bleached it white, everyone in New York freaked out. I didn't work for three months. Then I did the Valentino show in Paris. To do serious, proper frocks with a punk haircut was a big deal at the time. That suddenly made it okay. Everyone is scared to take a risk in New York. ■ I cut all my hair off because I just couldn't bear the hairdressers playing with it anymore. ■ I once had to meet Anthony Haden Guest at the Plaza Hotel for tea for an interview

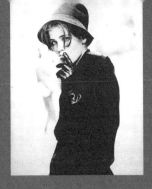

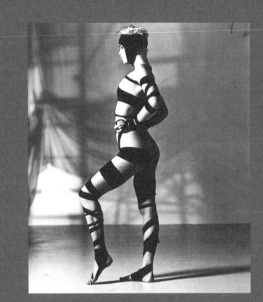

JENY
IS
THE
TYPE
WHO
WORE
TORN
JEANS
AND
DOC MARTENS
BEFORE
ANYONE
ELSE.

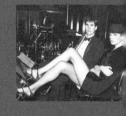

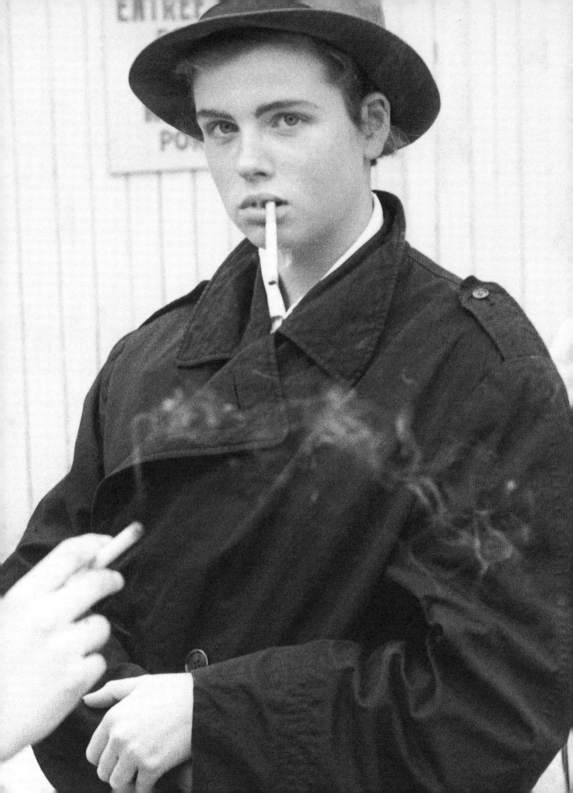

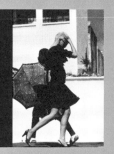

for *New York* magazine. The concierge wouldn't let me in because I had holes in my shoes. We ended up doing it outdoors. ■ I never knew what I wanted to do. The door just seemed to be open at the right time. I never had to try. I always seemed to be in the right place at the right time. If I had had to do go-sees like everyone else, I probably wouldn't have bothered. ■ Arthur was great because he liked me for myself, taught me how to bring out the best

On Money   I never had a boyfriend who made as much money as I did. They were always poor. I never met a rich guy I liked. I had a bloody good time throwing my money away. I look back and think, "Oh, my God, where did that ten grand go?" But I wouldn't have done it any other way.

What Modeling Taught Me   I learned how to get along with people — the high-strung, neurotic hairdresser and the editor whining about the right pair of earrings. I learned the hard way. You meet a lot of interesting people—and a lot of shitty ones, too.

How I Did What I Did   If you get a horrible dress to model, you try running around or hiking it up. Arthur used to tell me not to look in the mirror.

What I Thought About Fashion   My philosophy is being comfy—I'm a tomboy. I like men's suits, Comme des Garçons and Yohji Yamamoto. I often get mistaken for a boy. I always shopped for my loafers and oxfords at Brooks Brothers and the salesmen would always want to send me to the ladies' department. I also liked police shoes from Caldor on Long Island. I think men's shoes always make my legs look thinner. For someone who's not into fashion, I have a huge amount of clothes in my closet. I used to buy things and never wear them.

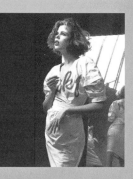

in myself. ■ I used to stay out all night and party—it's the only thing you have time to do. It was a release to go out and go mad. I never go out now. ■ Early on in New York, I'd get up in the morning and smoke a couple of joints. I could never do that now. ■ Once, I was supposed to be on location at six in the morning. I had been out all night and didn't get home until 7 A.M. I went straight to bed and unplugged the phone. But I learned my lesson—I got billed for everyone on the shoot."

"nudity.

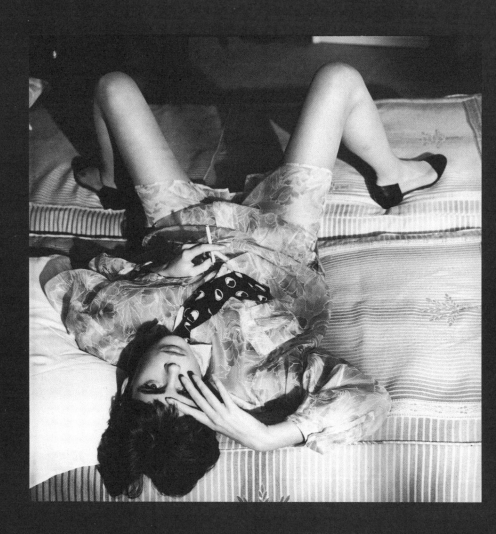

was never an issue for me. I always felt better when I didn't have any clothes on.

Besides, I hate wearing underwear."

How I Kept My Cool: Everyone has a different idea of success. I thought working steadily was being more successful than being a superstar one season, then burning out the next. Basically, you're there to sell a fucking dress and that's what it boils down to. I never took modeling seriously. It was not a childhood dream, so I did what I felt like.

The Future: I feel like modeling today has come full circle back to when I first started. It's gone through the glam, supermodel phase, and now it's back to grungy, boyish-looking girls. Really, I can't wait to be forty. I think that's when I'll be my best.

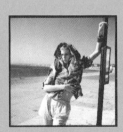

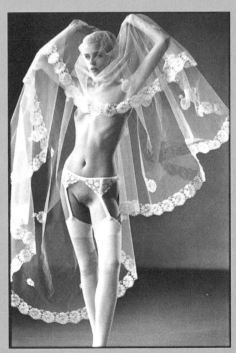

"I DON'T THINK OF MYSELF AS A STAR MODEL.

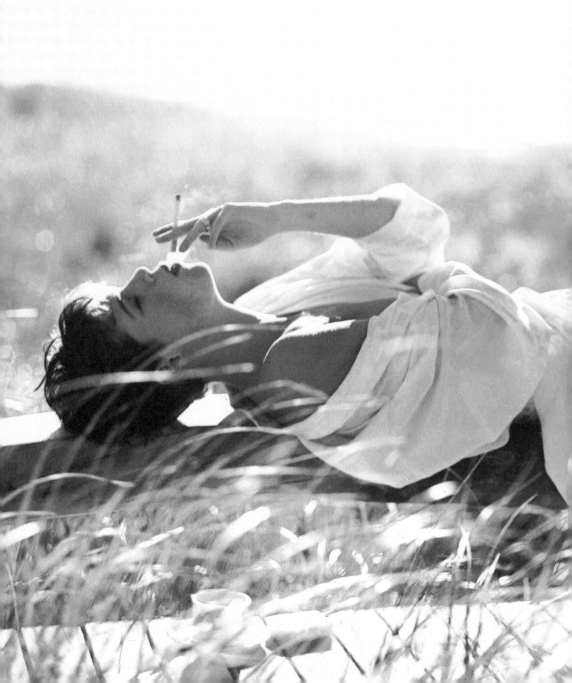

I COULD NEVER UNDERSTAND ALL THE FUSS."

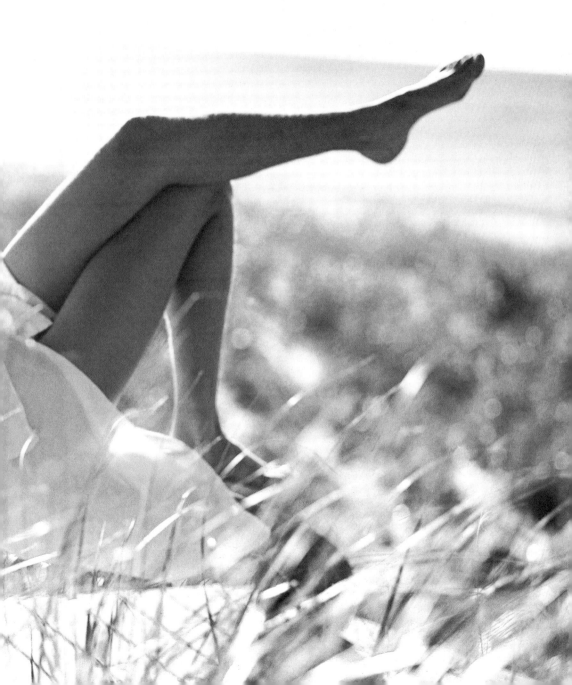

BAD
GIRL

"AMERICAN GIRLS ARE BROUGHT UP WITH THE IDEA OF
BEING RICH AND FAMOUS. ALL THEY WANT IS TEETH AND
HAIR. I WASN'T BROUGHT UP LIKE THAT. BEING A BRIT
ALLOWED ME TO GET AWAY WITH A WHOLE LOT MORE. I
GUESS I WAS KNOWN FOR BEING A REBEL AND A BAD GIRL,
BUT, REALLY, I WAS JUST BEING MYSELF. I WAS YOUNG AND
SELFISH AND DID WHAT I WANTED TO DO."

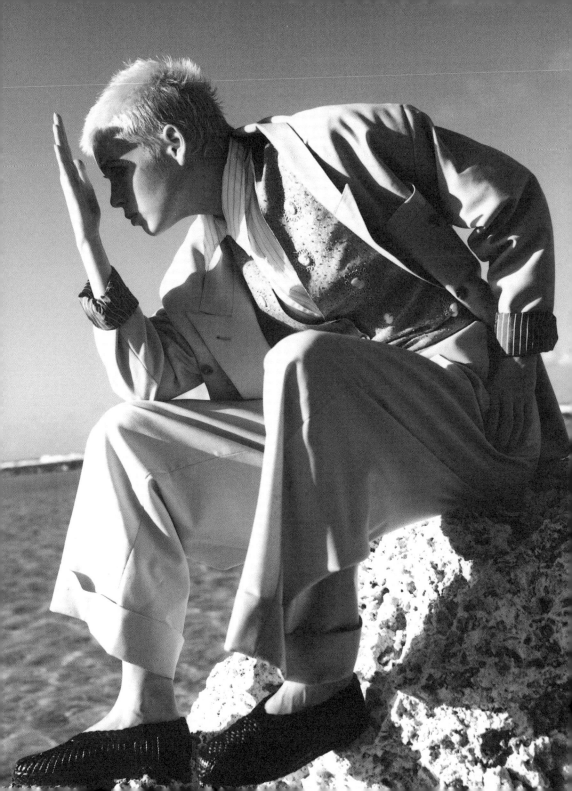

"I was just a scruffy, boyish punk from London."

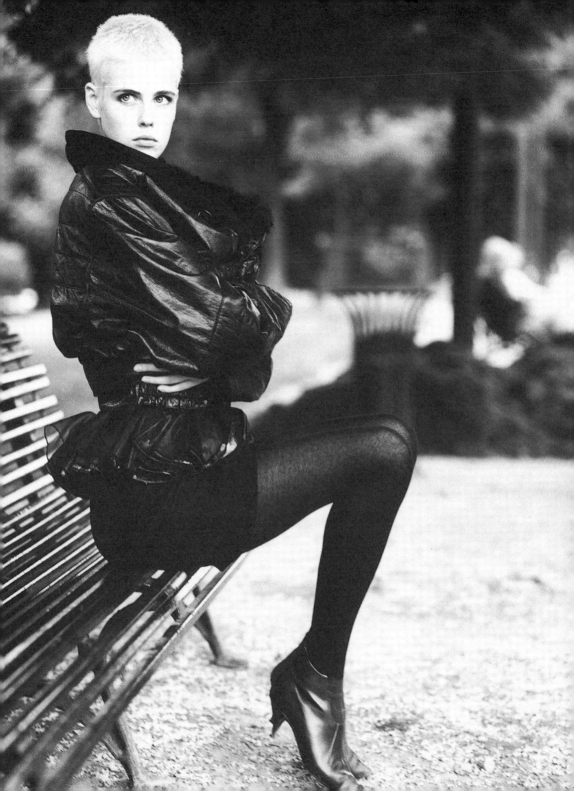

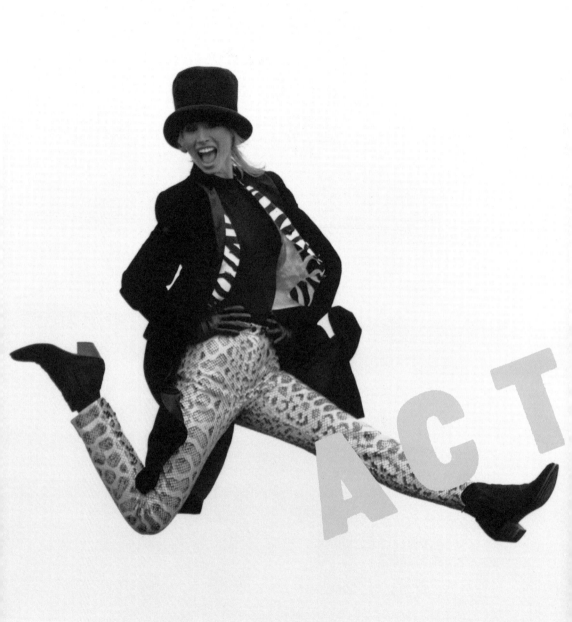

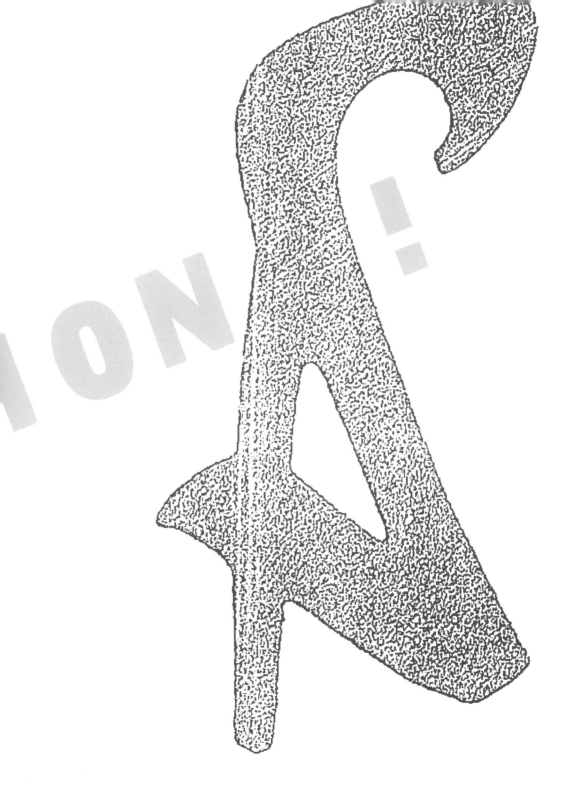

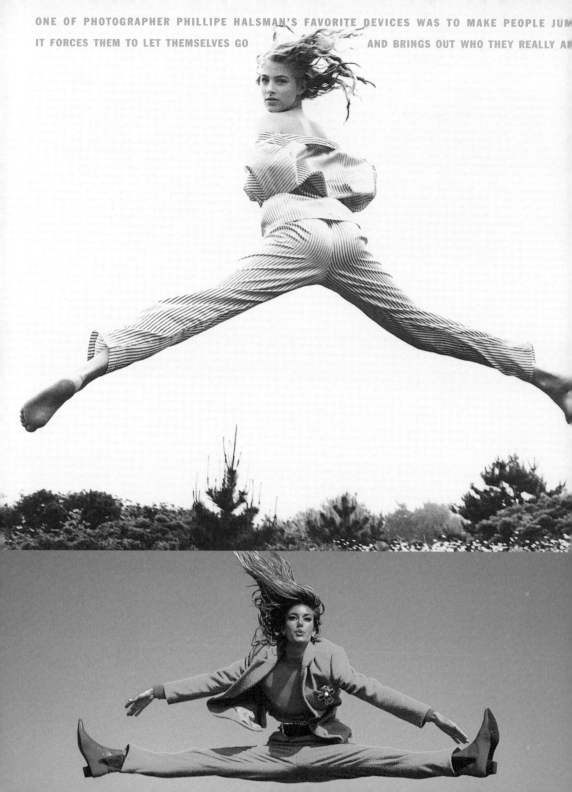

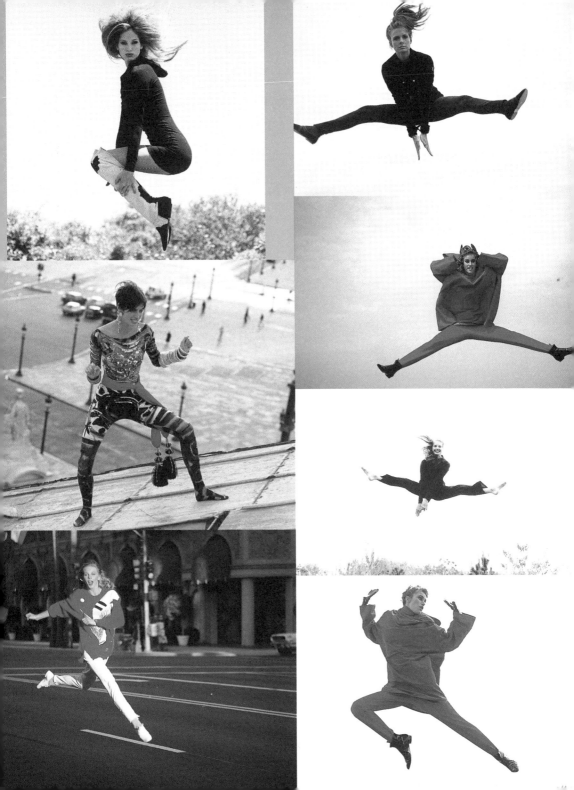

Posing in midair reminds me of dancing.

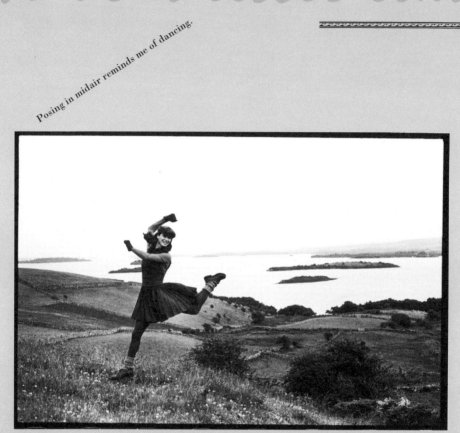

GRETHE HOLBY

Fashion and dance are both about face and body control.

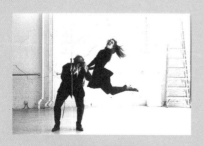

GRETHE AND ME

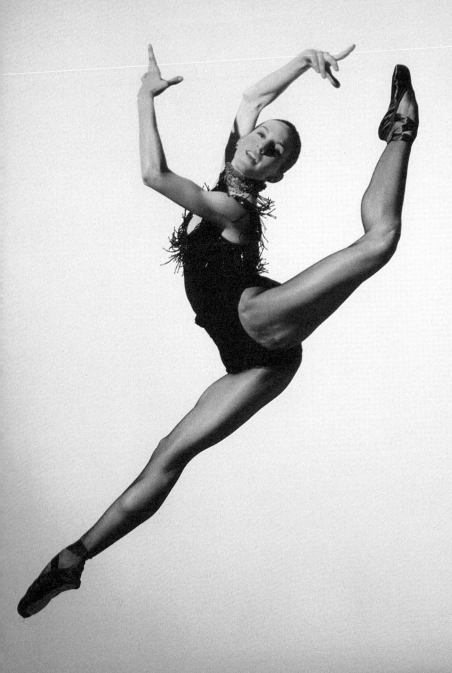

WENDY WHELAN

BODY

LANGUAGE

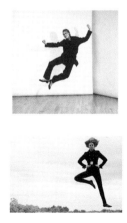

You start to realize very quickly what the difference is between a girl who is not just a lie-down-leaner but a girl who can really move. I like range — the one who can really negotiate any street, any staircase, any difficult situation. Especially when you have twenty pages of a story to do. A model needs to be supple and in charge of her body — she can't just sit there and be a pretty face.

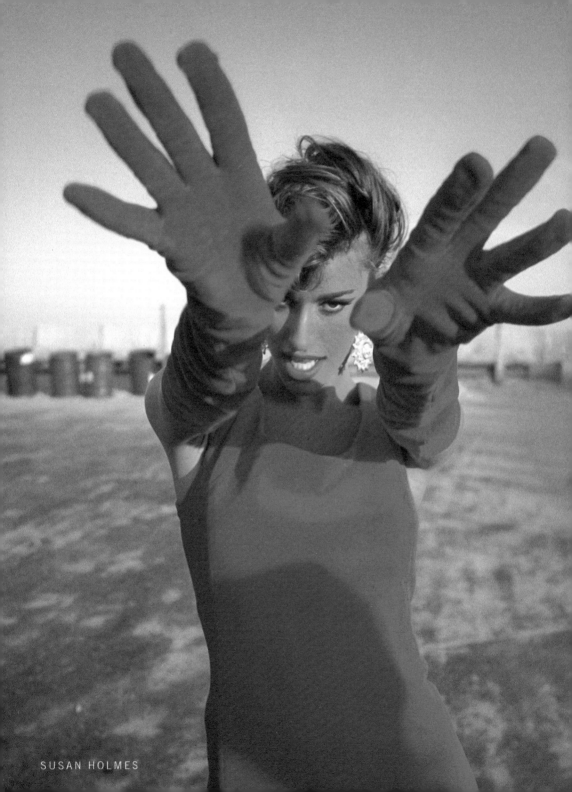

SUSAN HOLMES

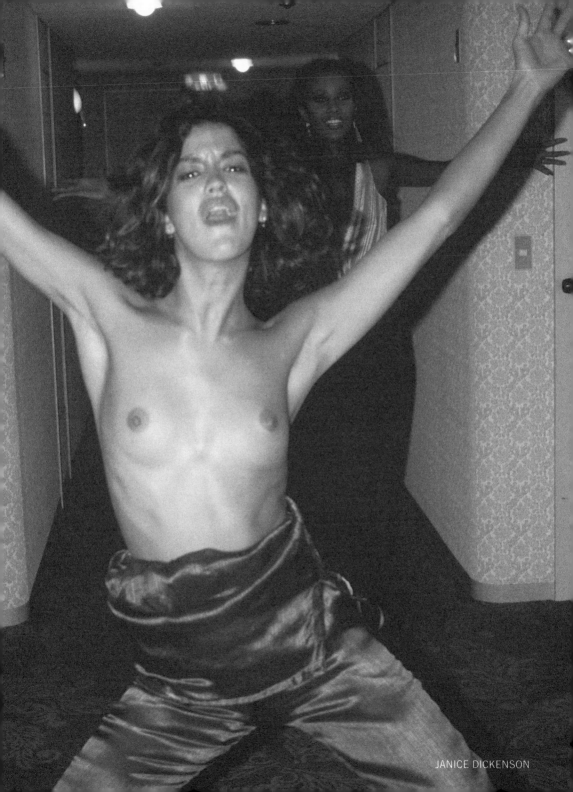

JANICE DICKENSON

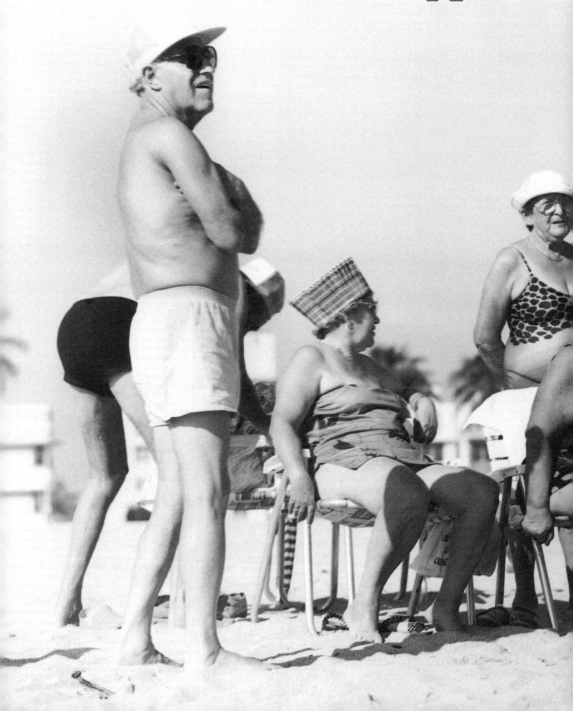

YOU ARE

NOT 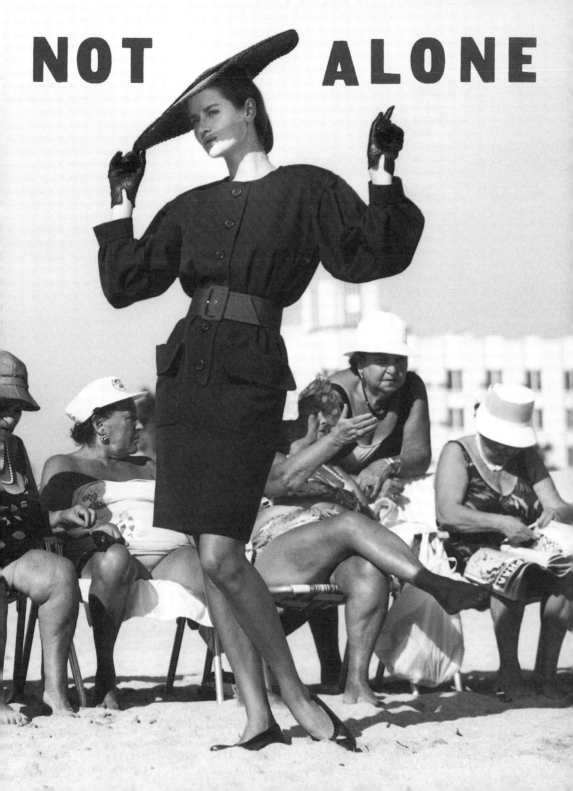 ALONE

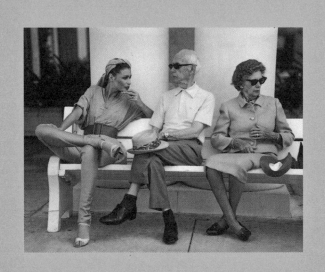

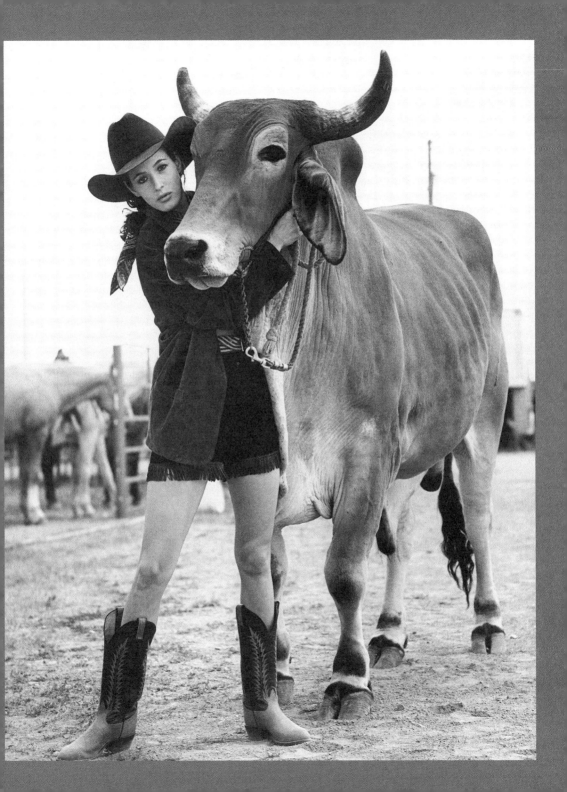

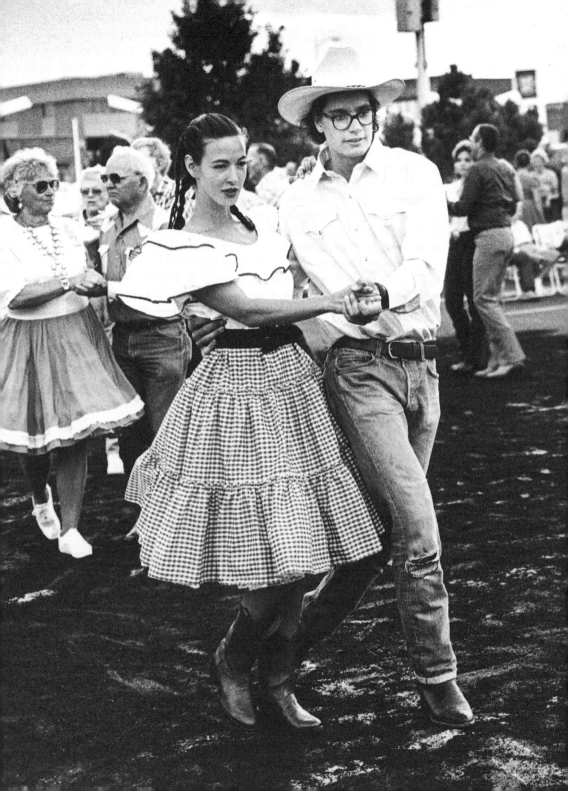

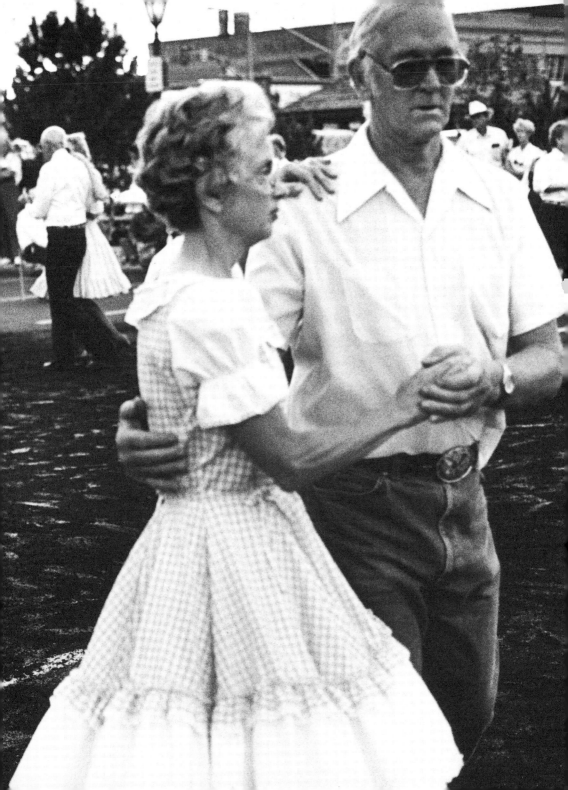

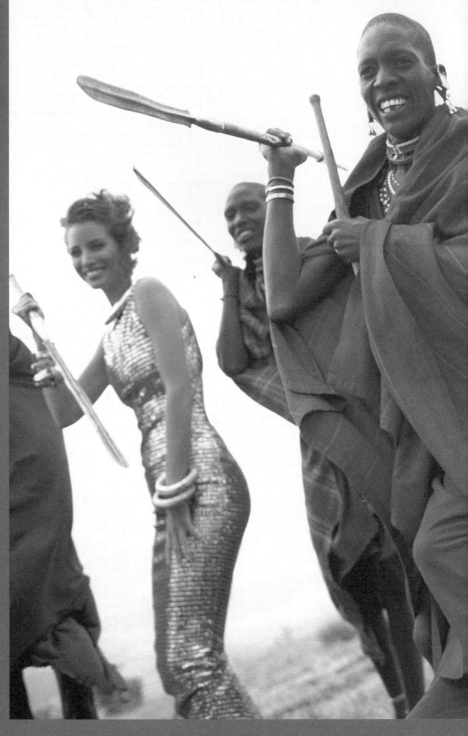

IF YOU'RE GOING TO BE A MODEL, YOU HAVE TO RELATE TO OTHERS WHEN YOU'RE ON A SHOOT.

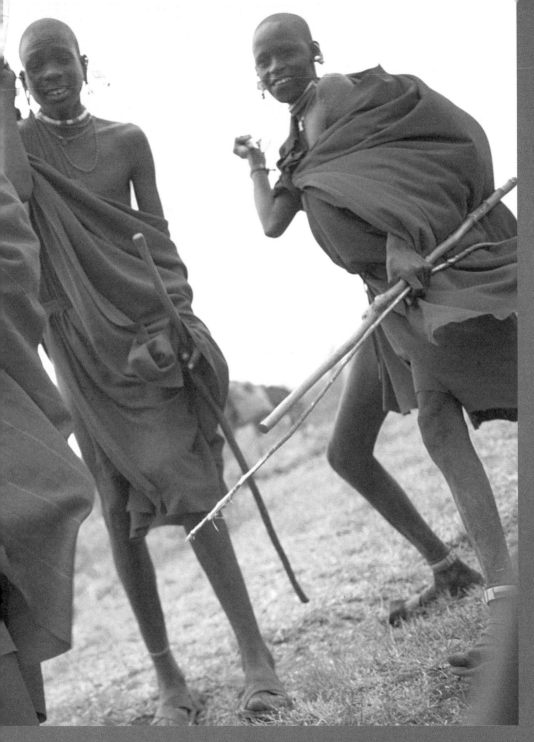

YOU NEED TO BE A LITTLE BIT OF A SOCIAL AMBASSADOR, TO EXPERIENCE THE PLACE.

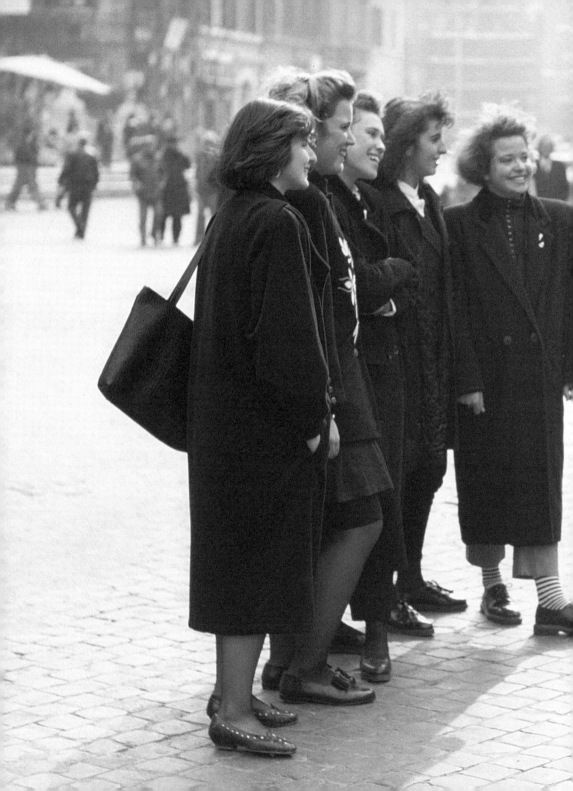

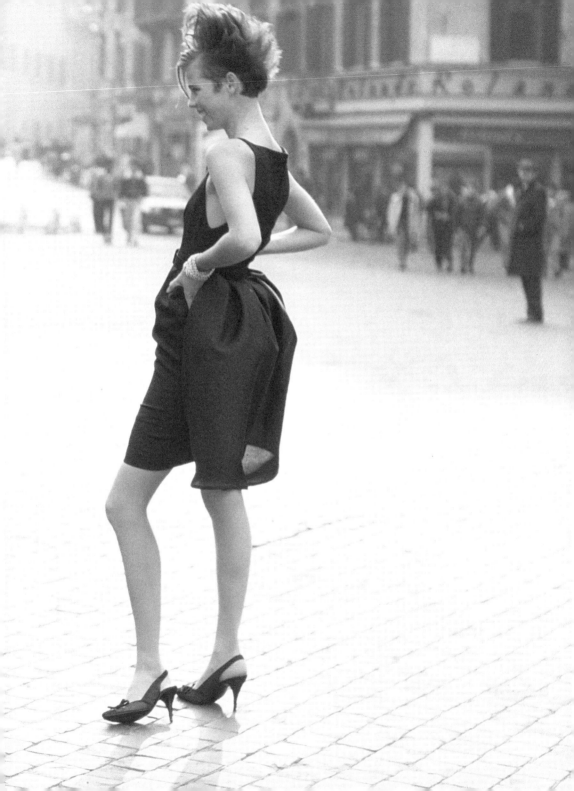

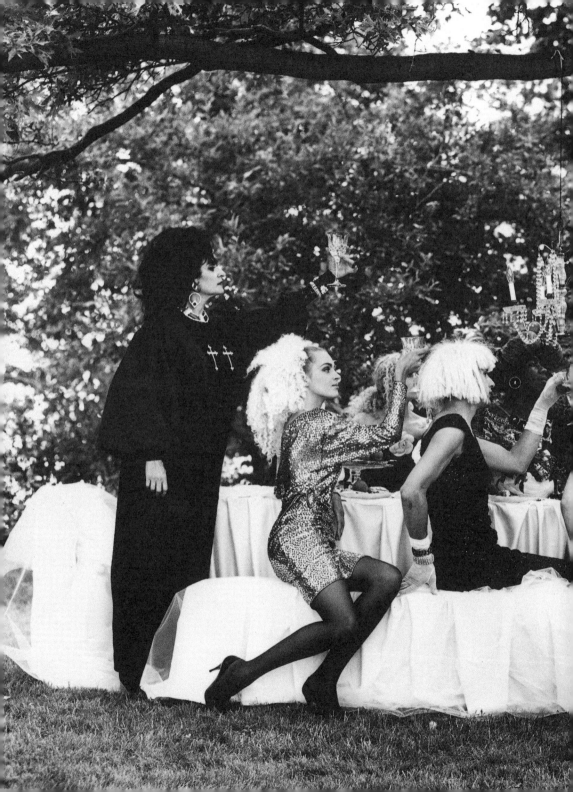

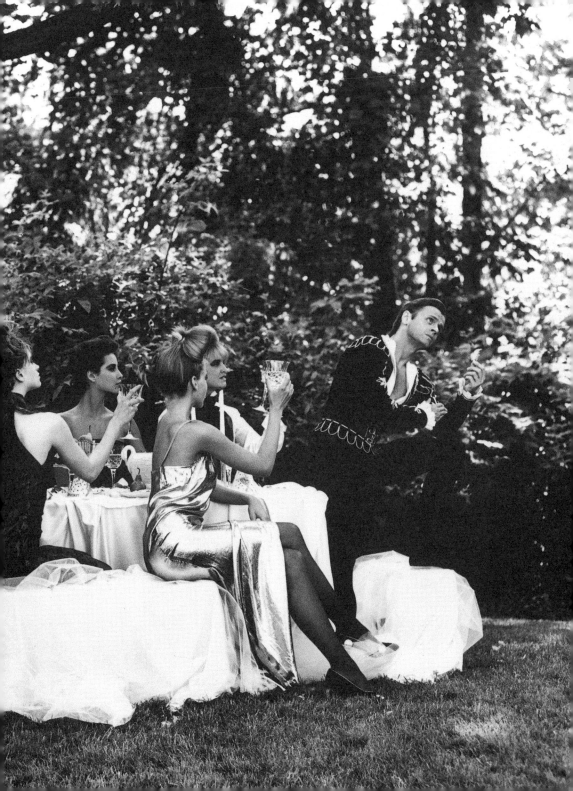

ALTHOUGH SOME OF THE TIME IT MIGHT JUST BE YOU IN FRONT OF THE CAMERA, THERE ARE PLENTY OF INSTANCES WHEN YOU ARE NOT ALONE—IT HELPS IF YOU CAN JUMP IN AND DO THE TWO-STEP AT A SQUARE DANCE OR CHAT IT UP ON THE BEACH WITH THE MIAMI LOCALS. IT'S A MATTER OF BEING LOOSE, OF INTERACTING WITH THOSE AROUND YOU SO THAT WE CAN GET THE BEST SHOT—EVEN IF YOU'RE JUST HAM-MING WITH A FEW MALE MODELS OR CUDDLING SOMEBODY'S SHARPEI.

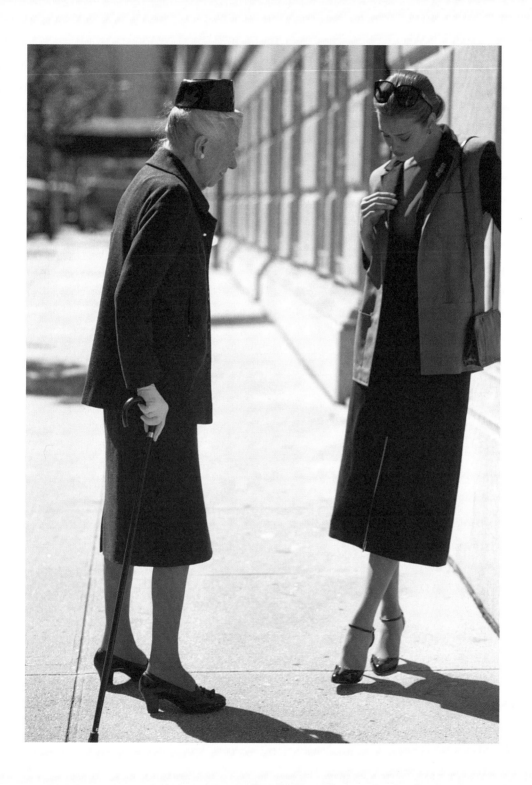

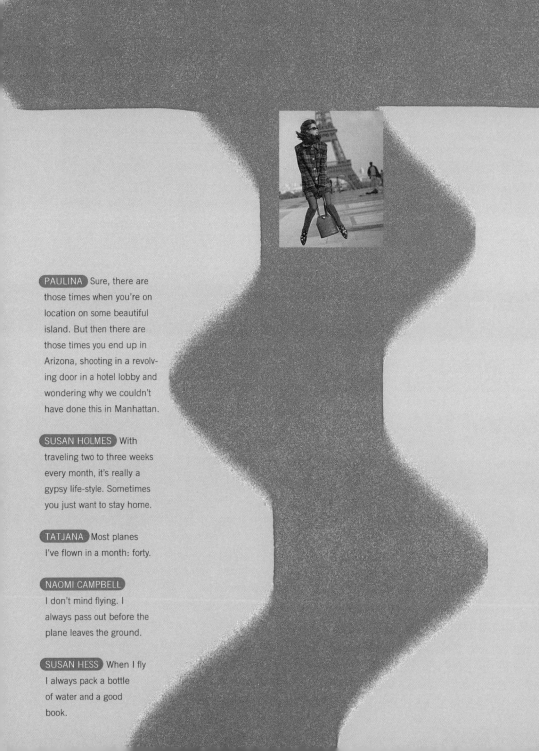

PAULINA Sure, there are those times when you're on location on some beautiful island. But then there are those times you end up in Arizona, shooting in a revolving door in a hotel lobby and wondering why we couldn't have done this in Manhattan.

SUSAN HOLMES With traveling two to three weeks every month, it's really a gypsy life-style. Sometimes you just want to stay home.

TATJANA Most planes I've flown in a month: forty.

NAOMI CAMPBELL I don't mind flying. I always pass out before the plane leaves the ground.

SUSAN HESS When I fly I always pack a bottle of water and a good book.

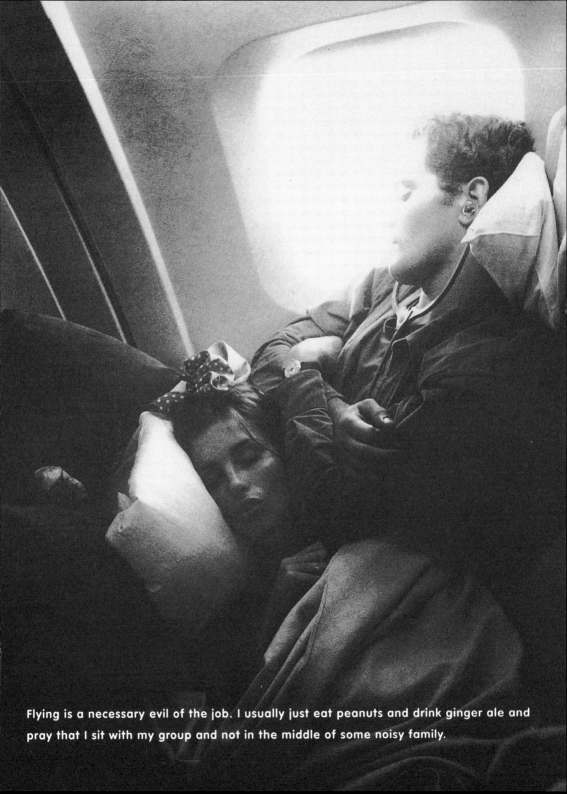

Flying is a necessary evil of the job. I usually just eat peanuts and drink ginger ale and pray that I sit with my group and not in the middle of some noisy family.

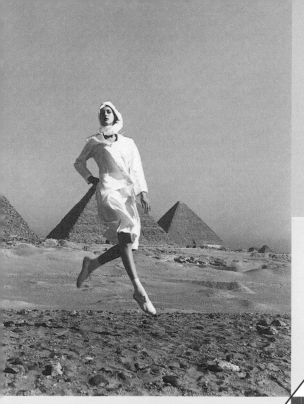

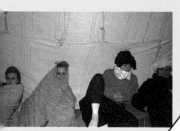

Early in the morning, before the
sun comes up and the
picture gets shot.

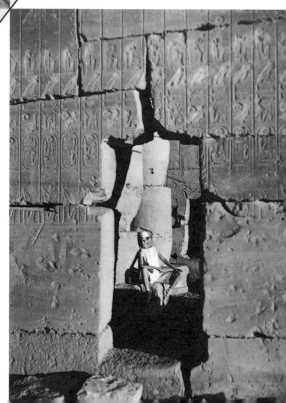

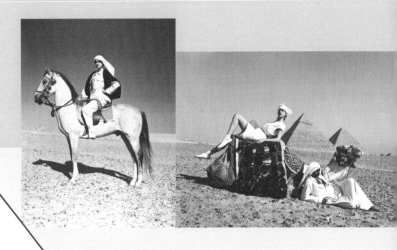

location work has its own set of rules:

the onlookers

the weather

the dirt

the light

the food

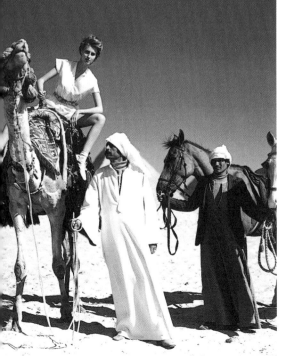

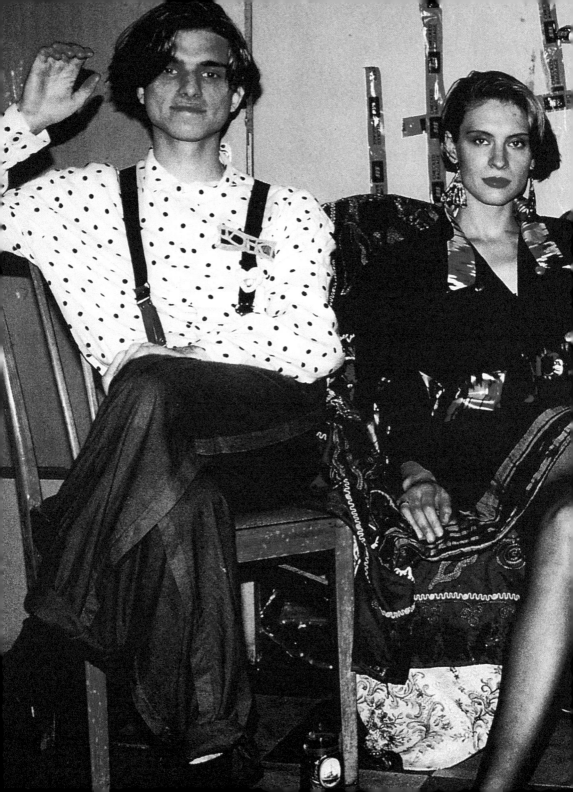

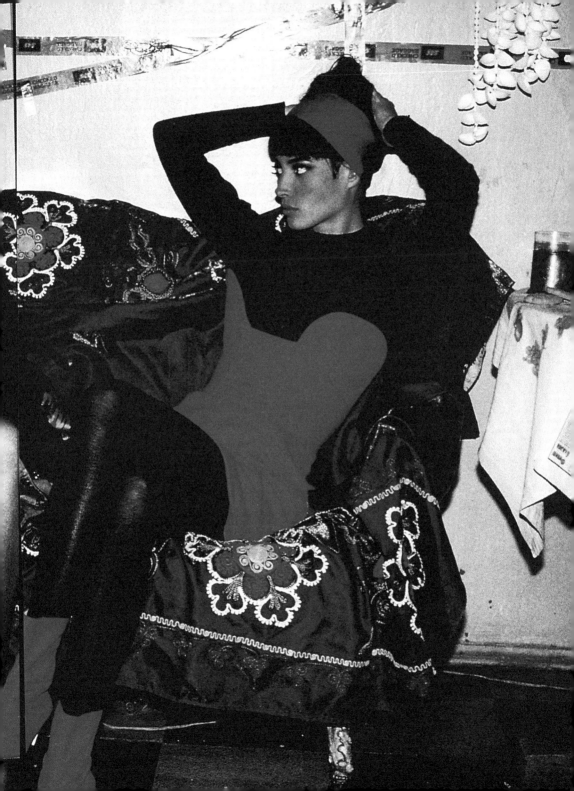

I LIKE A PICTURE THAT'S
INSPIRED BY REAL LIFE—A
WOMAN SITTING OUTSIDE AT A
CAFÉ TABLE, READING THE
PAPER AND DRINKING COFFEE.
I WANT TO WALK AWAY AND
COME BACK AND DISCOVER
THAT SAME SCENE WITH A
MODEL. I WANT TO GET THE
LOOK OF AN EAVESDROPPER.
IT'S ABOUT CREATING YOUR
OWN REALITY.

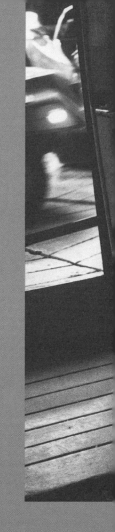

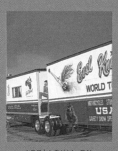

APOLLONIA ON
LOCATION
IN LAS VEGAS

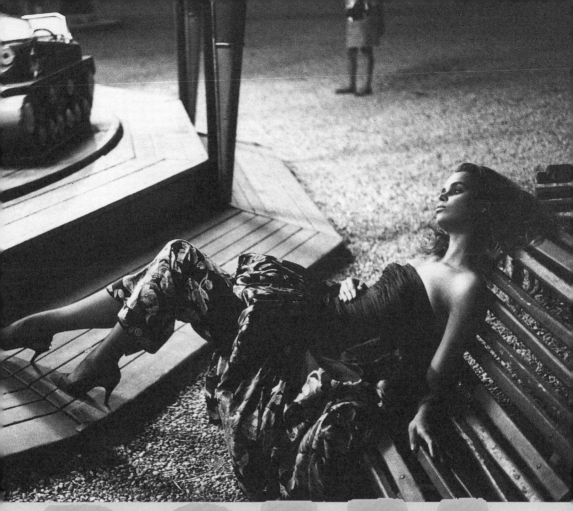

ROBYN MACKINTOSH

ROMA

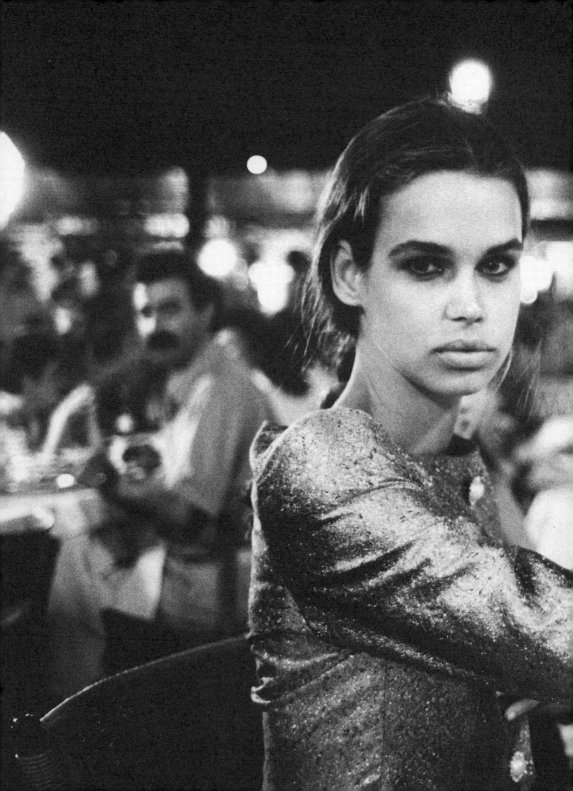

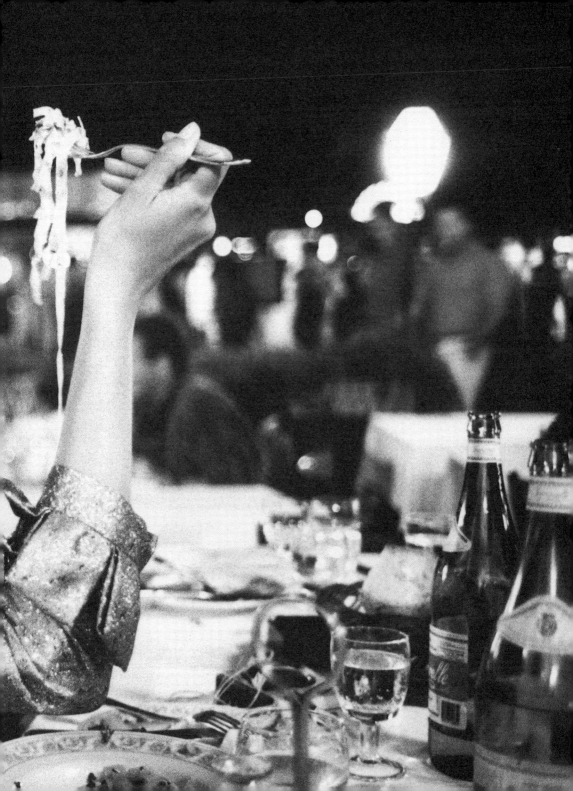

I STILL HAVE TO HOPE THAT
MY LUGGAGE ARRIVES, THE
PLANE TAKES OFF AND I
WILL GET THERE ON TIME.
WILL CUSTOMS IMPOUND MY
CAMERAS? WILL IT SNOW IN
SANTE FE WHEN IT'S SUP-
POSED TO BE SUNNY?

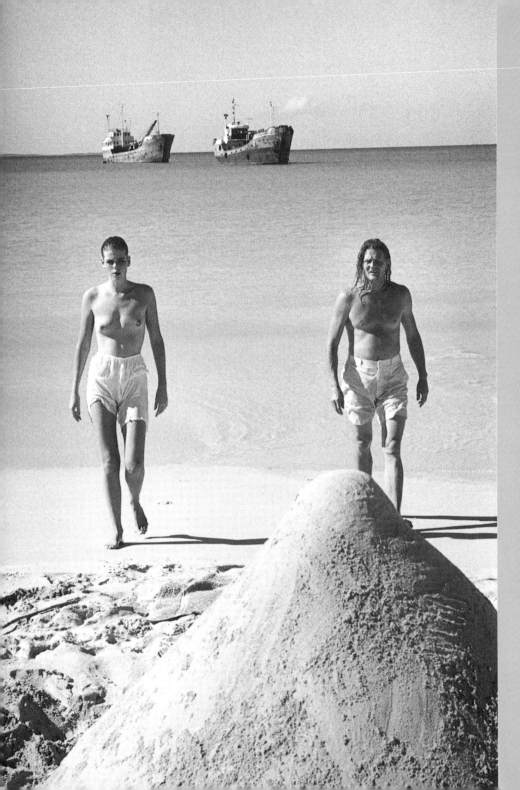

Jeny Howorth and Christiaan in Anguilla

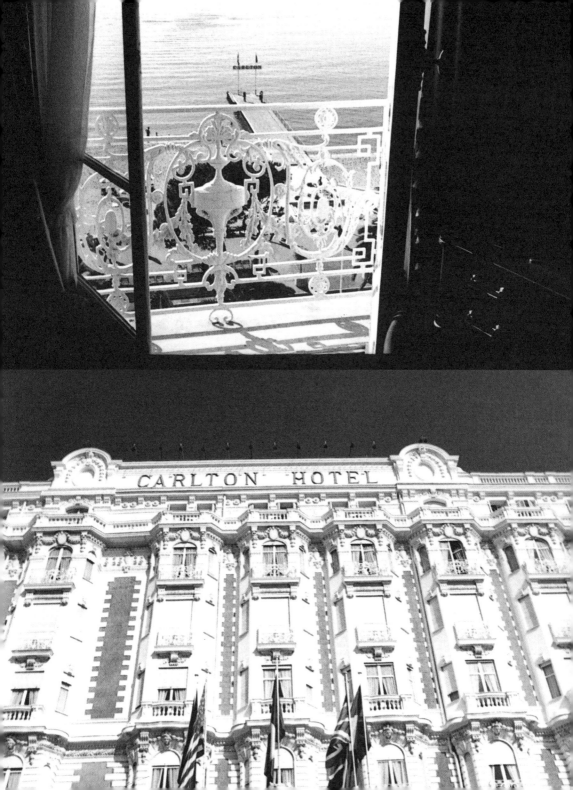

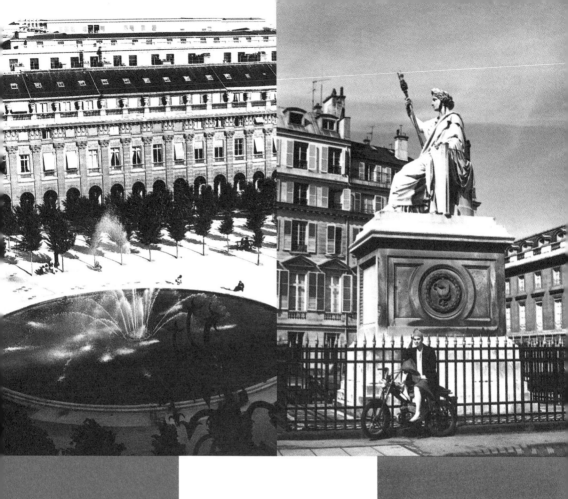

LINDA EVANGELISTA "WHEN I ARRIVE SOMEWHERE, I PRETEND THAT I'VE ALWAYS BEEN THERE."

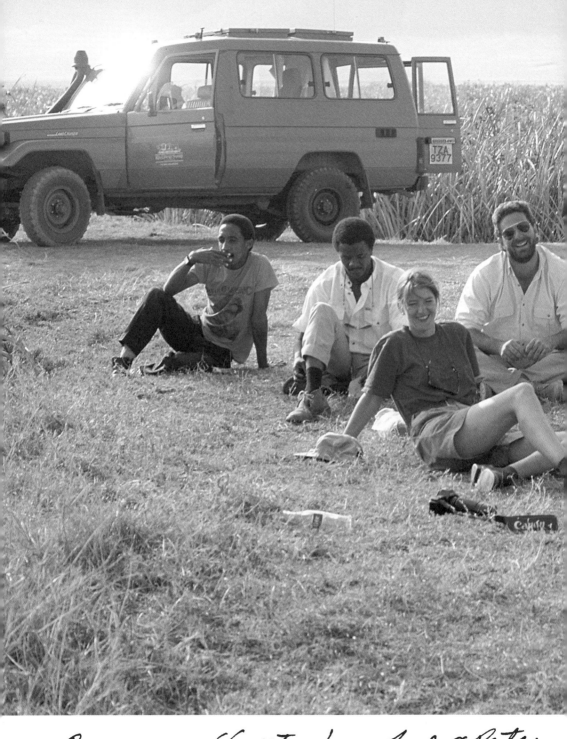

Our gang Christy Sara Jane & Peter

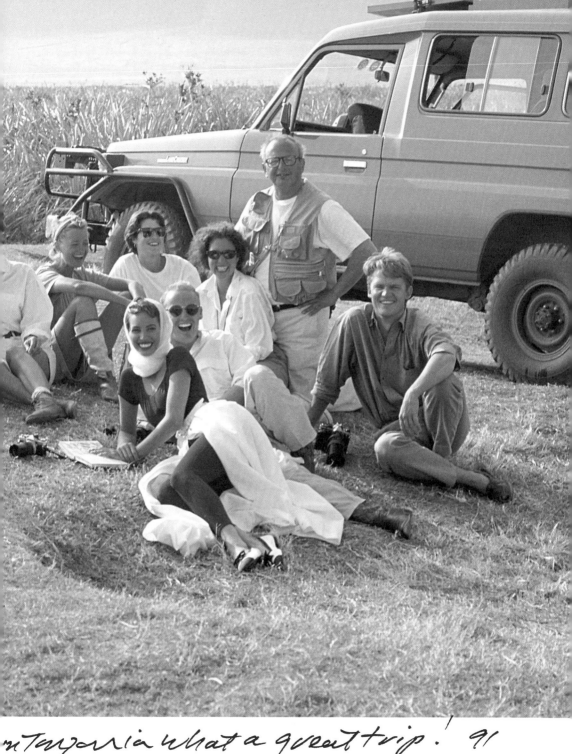

n Tanzania what a great trip! 91

We get to travel the way a tourist doesn't. We get to be insiders. On a four-day shoot at a private home in Scotland, we get to see what the snooker room and the kitchen are like.

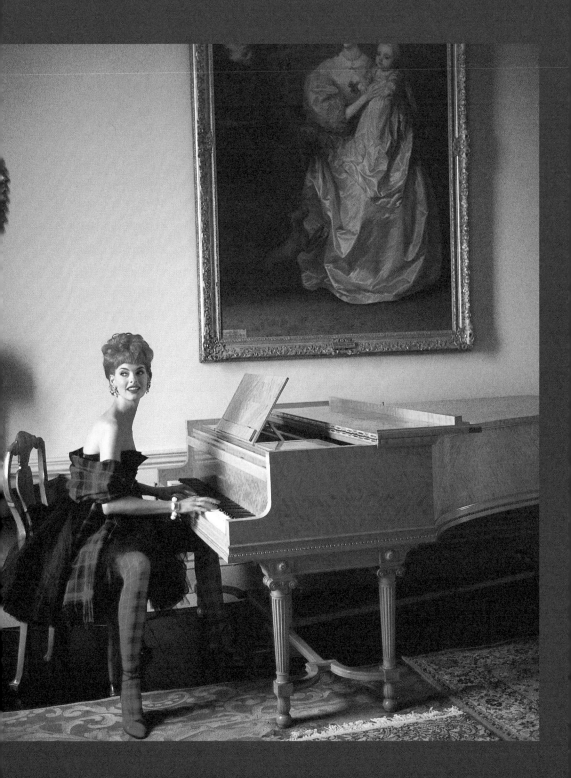

Patti was

My Fair Lady

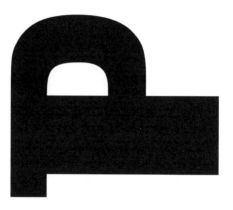

from

Staten Island

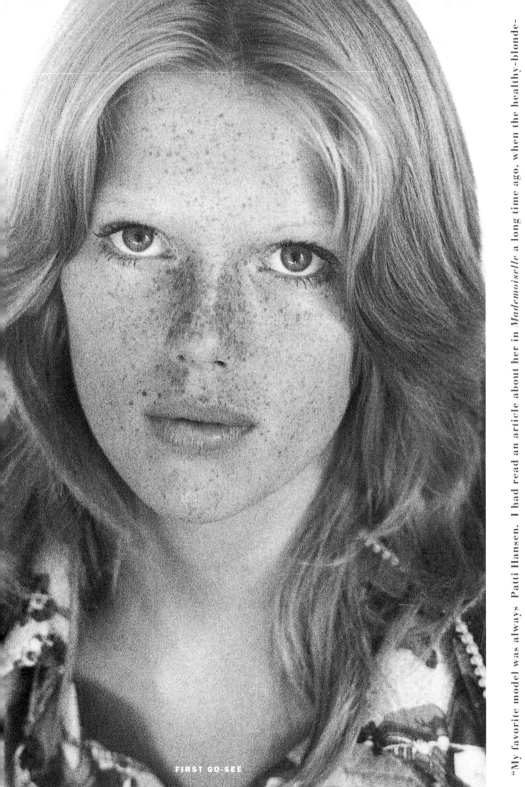

"My favorite model was always Patti Hansen. I had read an article about her in *Mademoiselle* a long time ago, when the healthy-blonde-model look was in. She told how she was happiest staying home, stuffing her face with pizza. I totally related to that." —Jeny Howorth

FIRST GO-SEE

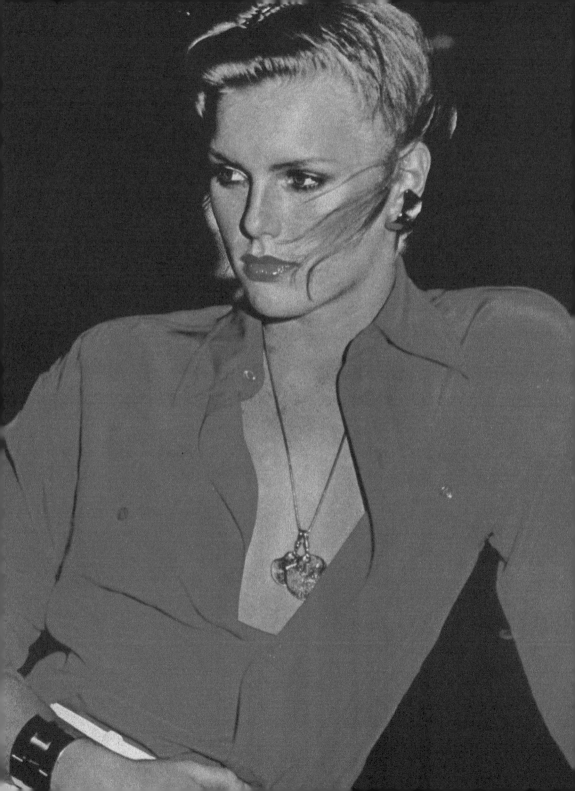

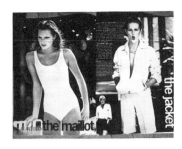

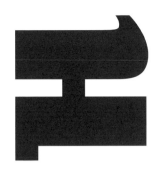

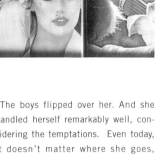

When she first came to see me, I thought she looked like a nice neighborhood girl, clean and regular. At our first shoot together for Geoffrey Beene, Polly [Mellen] put ridiculously high heels on her. Of course, she couldn't take a step without tripping, so Polly arranged to have her take them home with her so she could practice walking. Polly wanted her to slim down, so she said, "Now I don't want you to eat anything for a while." For her first *Vogue* cover shoot, she wore a low-cut shirt that brought out the Marilyn Monroe in her. Suddenly she was no longer the girl next door.

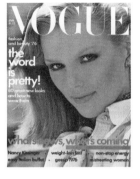

"The boys flipped over her. And she handled herself remarkably well, considering the temptations. Even today, it doesn't matter where she goes, nothing has changed. She looks so extraordinary the men are still whistling and trying to pick her up. Most of the time it's her own fault—she just loves a good-looking guy. I think she just has that animal thing...."

—Polly Mellen

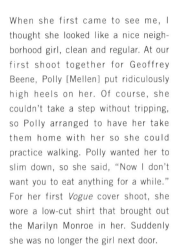

I remember the phone ringing and Polly Mellen, then at *Vogue*, was on the line, saying, "Arthur, I have someone *sooo* wonderful to send to you. She's a beauty—you'll love her." And I did.

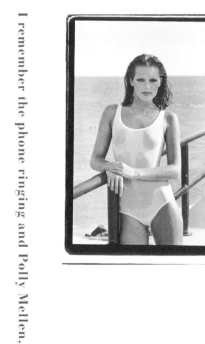

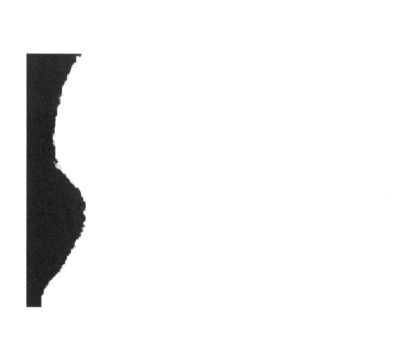

susan

hess

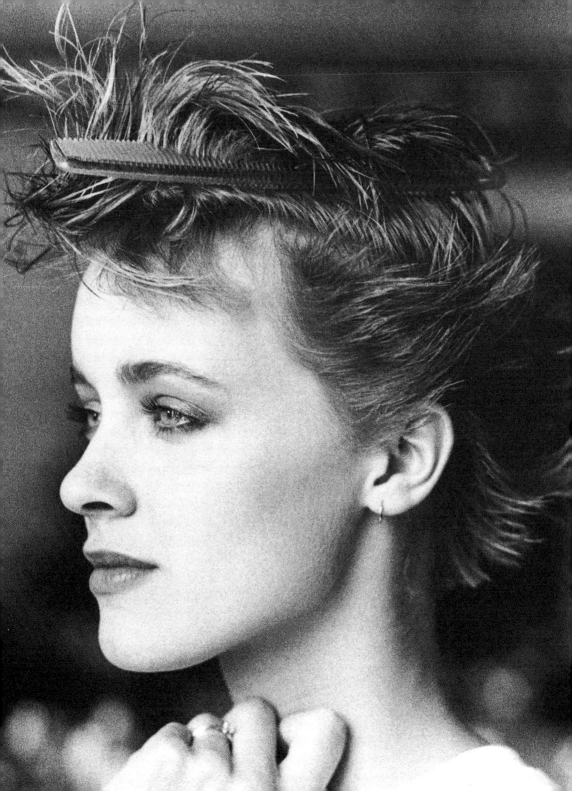

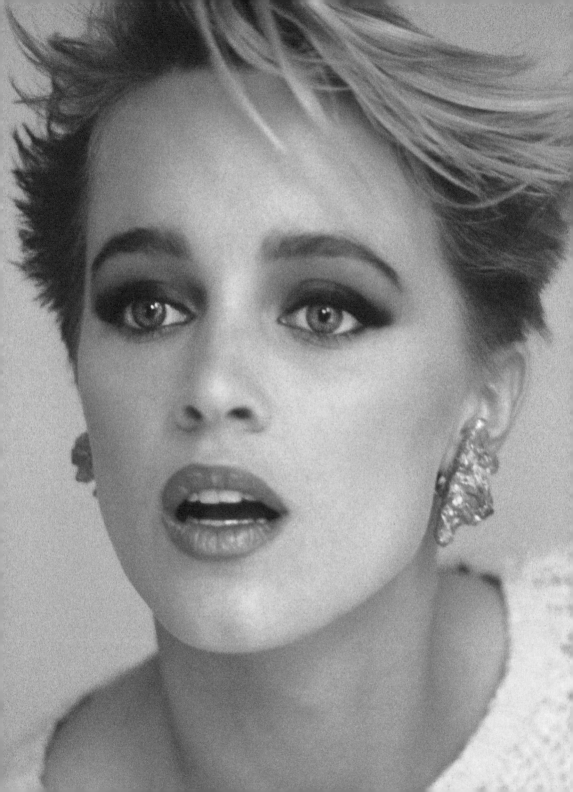

Certain girls...

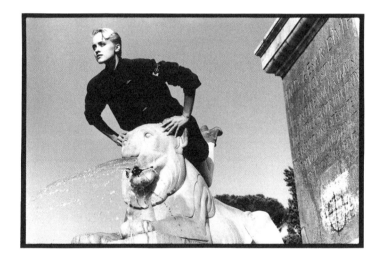

...can make a picture happen. You don't have to draw them out. Susan was very aware of presentation, of making herself better for the camera. She could walk, she could run, she could act. She was intuitive.

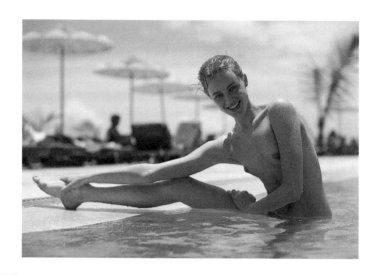

"I was always aware...

...of breathing and posture when I was having my picture taken. I would try to have a fantasy in my head. I had an idea of what the person being photographed would be doing and thinking. Then I'd create a persona through the clothes and try to maintain that character. To stand there and just look pretty never worked for me. When I was modeling, there was less of a conception of models as clotheshorses. The clothes were always an excuse to take the picture."

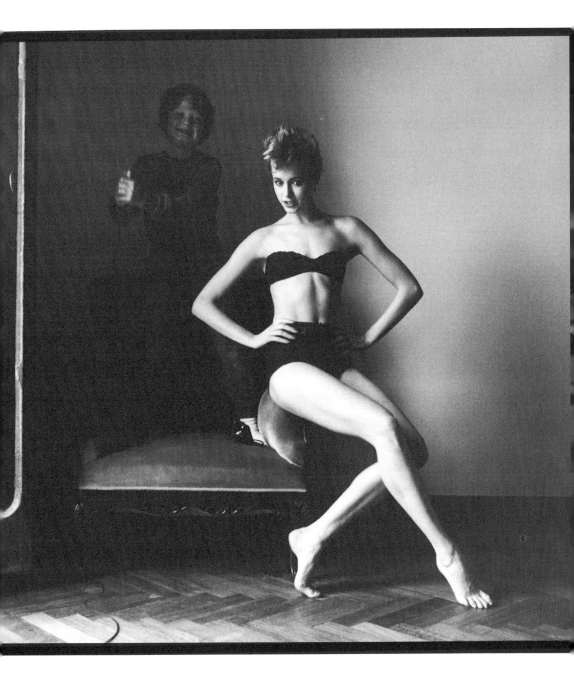

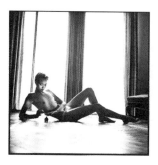

"I got into modeling because I wanted to be an actress. At about twenty-five, I started to see there wasn't much more for me to do. I'd kind of saturated the market. At any moment you knew your modeling career could be over. And when it did stop, it wouldn't be because you forgot how to pose. It would be because you weren't pretty enough or you were too old or they were bored with you. I knew it was time to stop.

At the peak of my career, I had a breast-implant operation. I looked at the acting world and decided women who succeeded in that field had a particular shape. I thought if I wanted to make it, I'd better improve my chances. At the time, no one in the modeling business had had the operation. I was horrified that someone would find out, but after I'd had mine everybody suddenly went for it. I was never comfortable with my breast implants, and in the end I developed severe health problems. Two years ago, I had them removed and wrote a magazine article about it. By coming out publicly, I risked being associated with the issue and, as a consequence, losing work. I made my peace with that choice, but it has taken me more than nine years to get over the feeling of not being pretty enough, not being good enough for anything, and so much of that came from modeling."

I love the way she moved. I loved her energy.

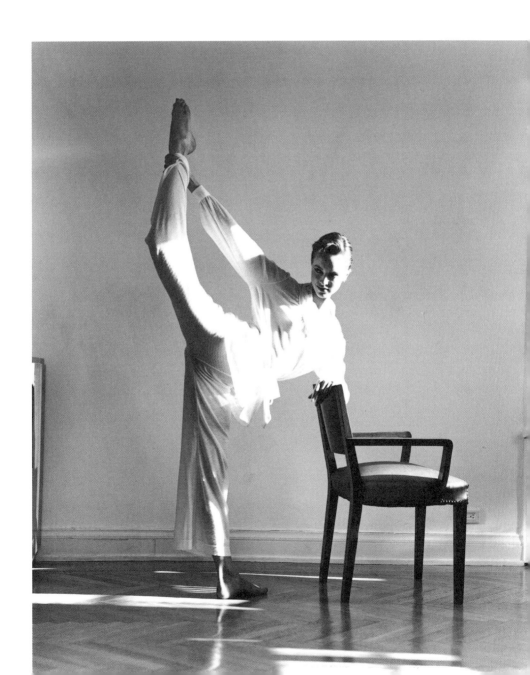

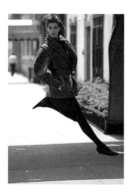

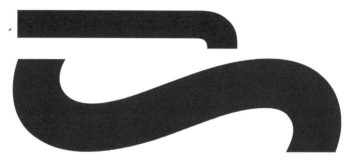

JOAN SEVERANCE

WE WERE SHOOTING COATS FOR AMERICAN *VOGUE* IN JULY. IT WAS HORRIBLY HOT. I HATED THE CLOTHES. I COULDN'T GET INTO IT. ALL I COULD THINK ABOUT WAS GETTING A JOB WITH A BEACH LOCATION. THEN JOAN STEPPED OUT OF THE VAN AND LOOKED AT ME. SHE WAS SO DAMNED STRIKING.

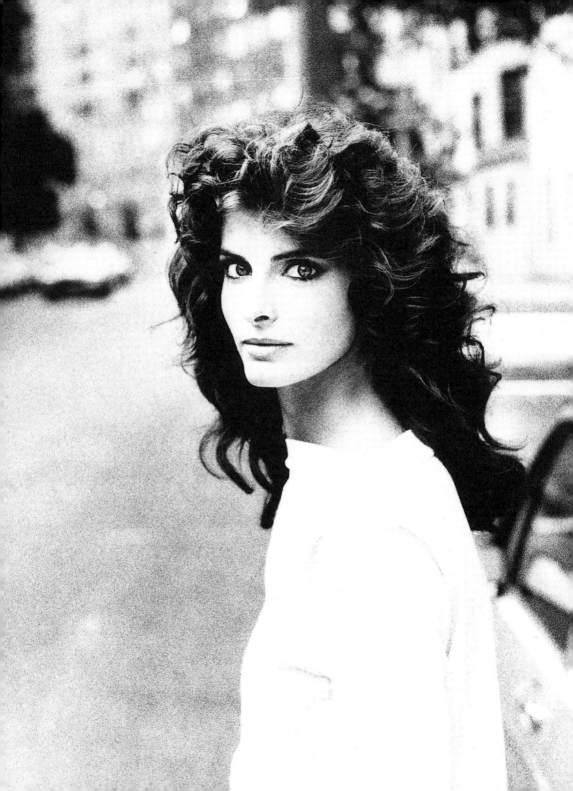

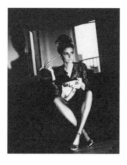

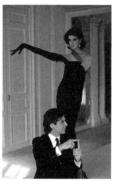

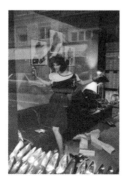

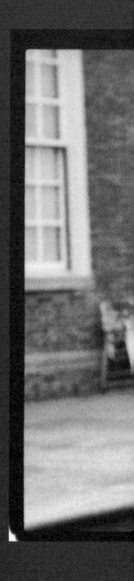

"MY ADVICE TO ASPIRING MODELS: YOU'D BETTER REALIZE THAT THERE ARE BILLIONS OF
BEAUTIFUL GIRLS. THERE WILL BE OBSTACLES THAT HAVE NOTHING TO DO WITH YOU."

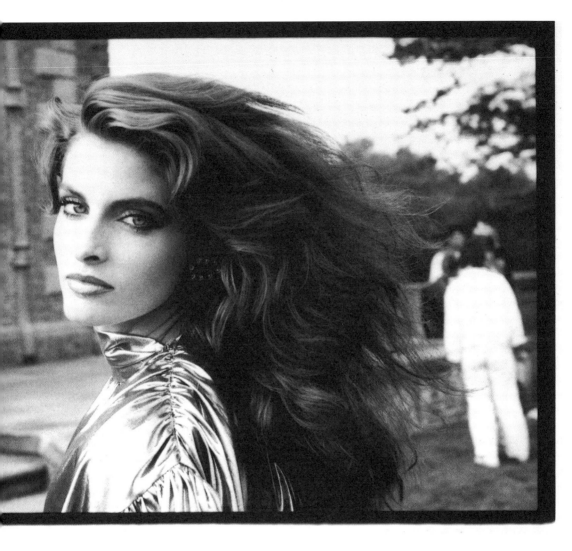

"I'M FROM HOUSTON. I STARTED MODELING IN 1974 TO MAKE MONEY

FOR COLLEGE. I QUIT IN 1984. IT GOT TO THE POINT THAT THE MONEY

JUST WASN'T IMPORTANT ANYMORE. I DID THINGS BACKWARDS—I

MADE A FORTUNE DOING COMMERCIAL WORK BEFORE I DID EDITORIAL.

I LOST EVERY MODELING CONTEST I EVER ENTERED."

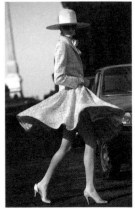

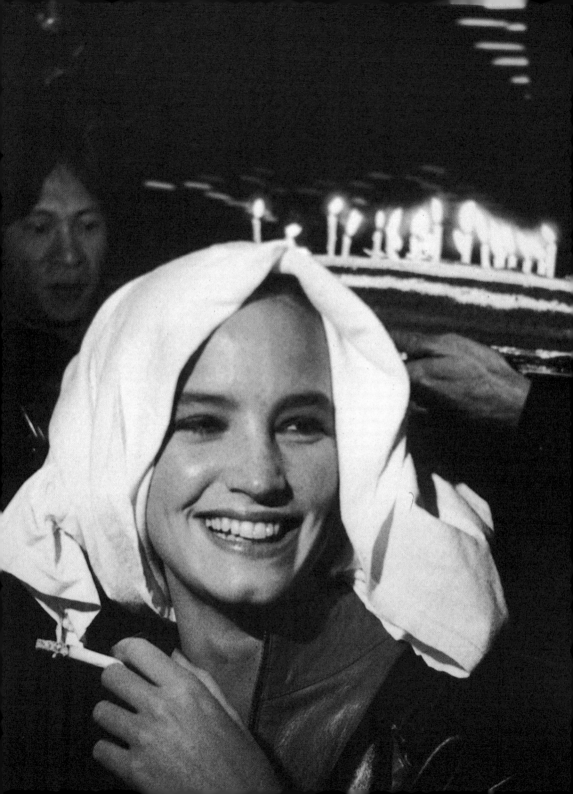

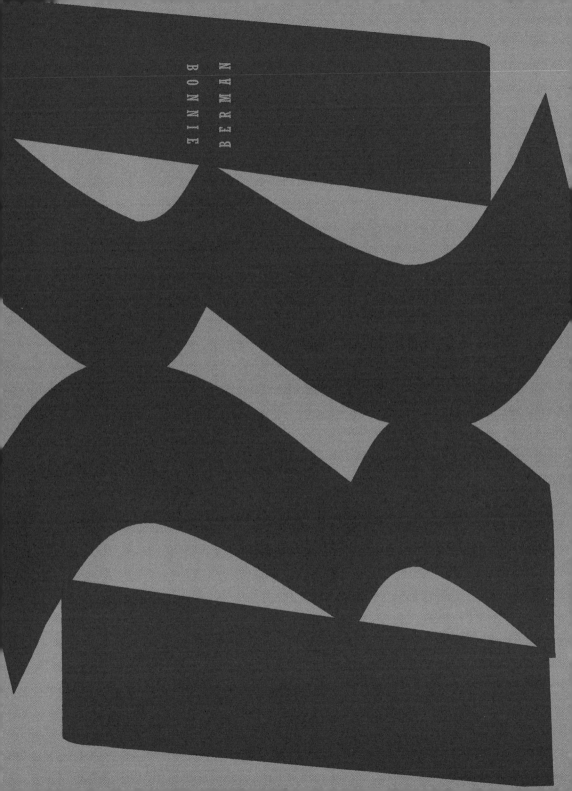

BONNIE BERMAN

BEAUTY

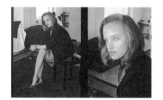

FIRST GO-SEE

"I ALWAYS FELT I WAS KIND OF STRANGE-LOOKING—NOT
PHYSICALLY PERFECT OR EVEN GLAMOROUS. BUT I CAME TO
MODELING AT AN INTERESTING TIME. IT WAS 1982 AND
THINGS WERE MOVING AWAY FROM THE FINE-BONED HALSTON
TYPES—THE JERRY HALL, JOAN SEVERANCE ERA.
SO THERE WAS THIS SENSE OF REVOLUTION, BUT A NEW LOOK
HADN'T BEEN CHOSEN. EDITORS AND PHOTOGRAPHERS WERE
EXPERIMENTING, WHICH I THINK HAD SOMETHING TO DO WITH
MY SUCCESS. I'M SORT OF FRESH-FACED. I HAD A LOT OF
FRECKLES AND THIS SANDY-BLONDE HAIR."

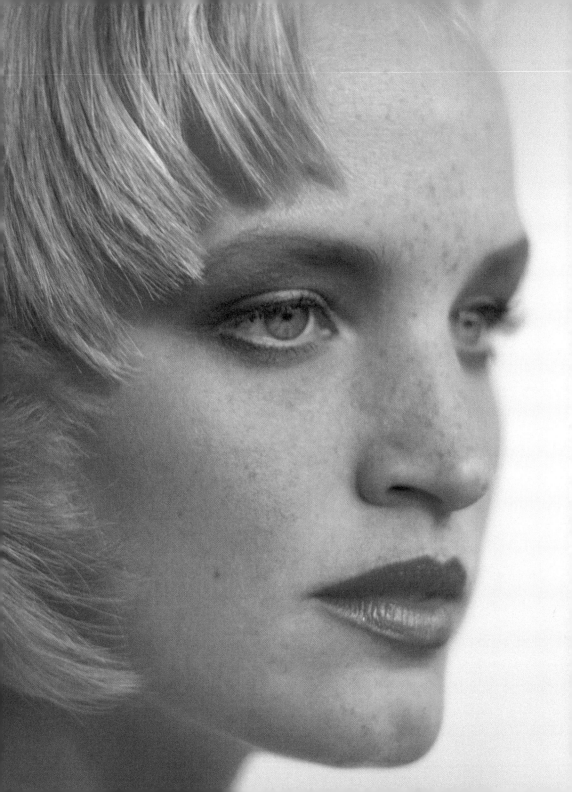

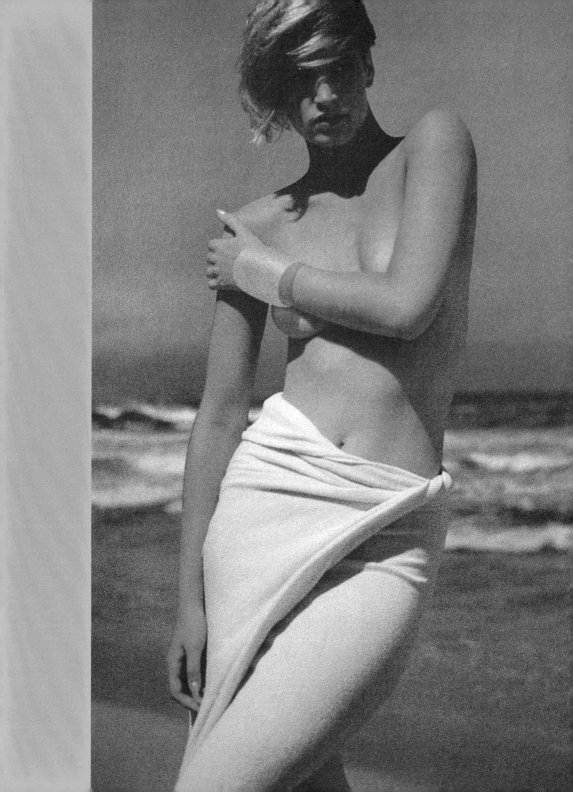

BODY

"I learned from the illustrator Antonio how to manage my body. What matters as much as your expression is the angles you create with your body... how to subconsciously break up space. I always had an idea of what I was doing.... Sometimes I'd think about poetry or use my imagination to generate a mood."

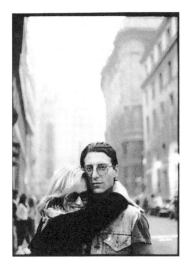
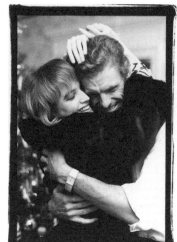
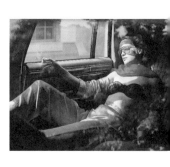

B R A

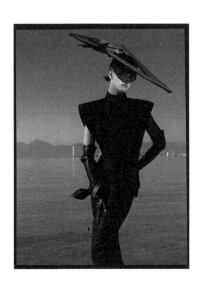
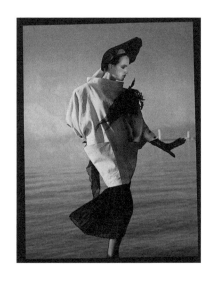

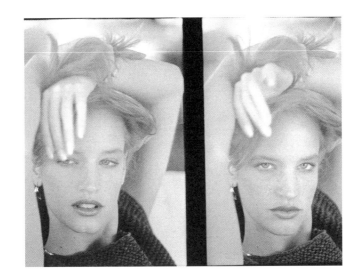

INS

"I WAS NOT VERY FASHION-MINDED. I ALWAYS HAD THIS QUIRKY STYLE.

I CAME INTO ARTHUR'S STUDIO THE FIRST DAY WEARING A 1930S THRIFT-SHOP SKIRT

AND A WORLD WAR I VEST. ARTHUR CALLED IT THE 'EASTERN EUROPEAN WAITRESS

LOOK.' WHEN I ENTERED MODELING THERE WEREN'T MANY GIRLS WITH PRINCETON

DEGREES. BUT ALL THE MODELS I'VE MET WHO ARE SUCCESSFUL ARE INTELLI-

GENT. THEY MAY NOT BE COLLEGE-EDUCATED, BUT THEY'RE ALL SMART."

✪

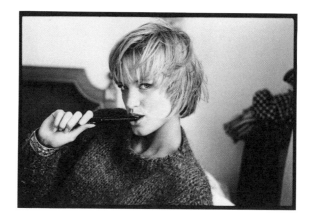

✪

CERTAIN GIRLS ARE NOT NECESSARILY BEAUTIFUL, BUT EVERYTHING FALLS IN

SUCH A WAY THAT YOU CAN PUT ANYTHING ON THEM. BONNIE WAS SUCH A GIRL.

SHE HAD INTELLIGENCE AND EXPRESSION. SHE WAS SAVVY AND PERSONAL,

AND I SAW THE BEAUTY IN HER.

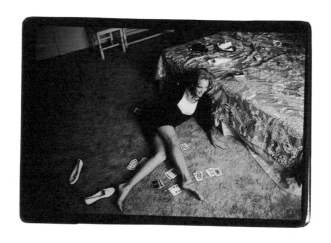

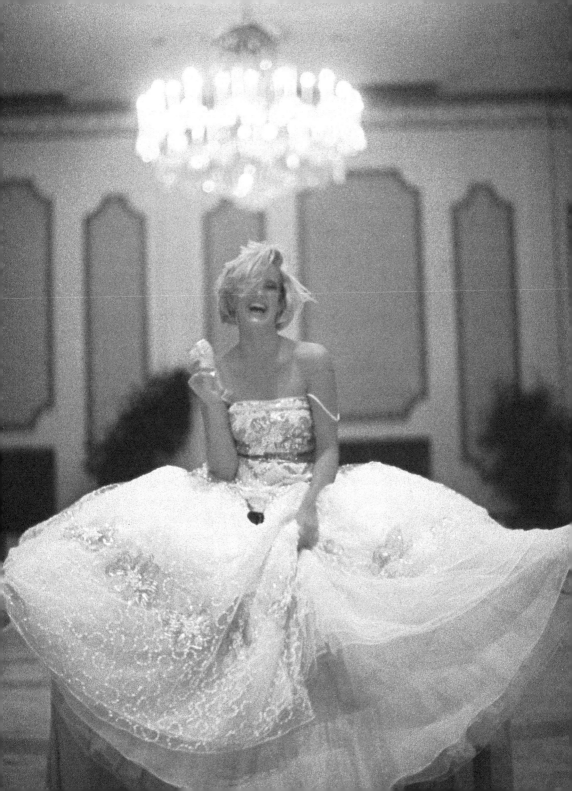

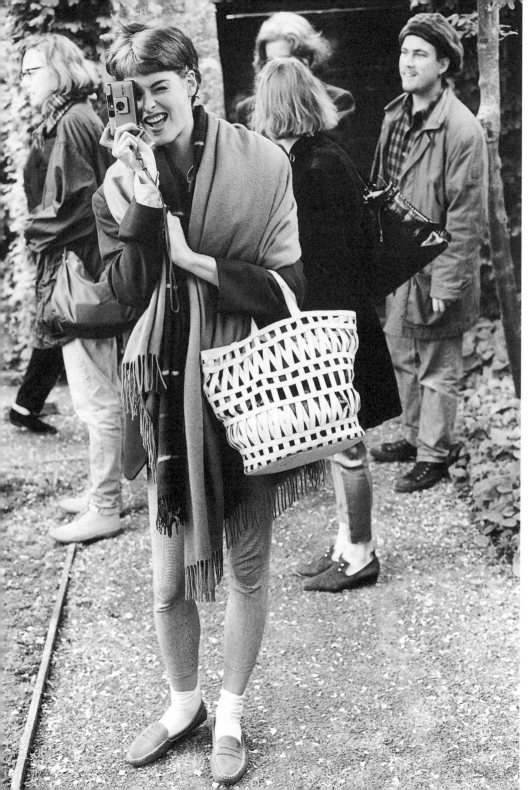

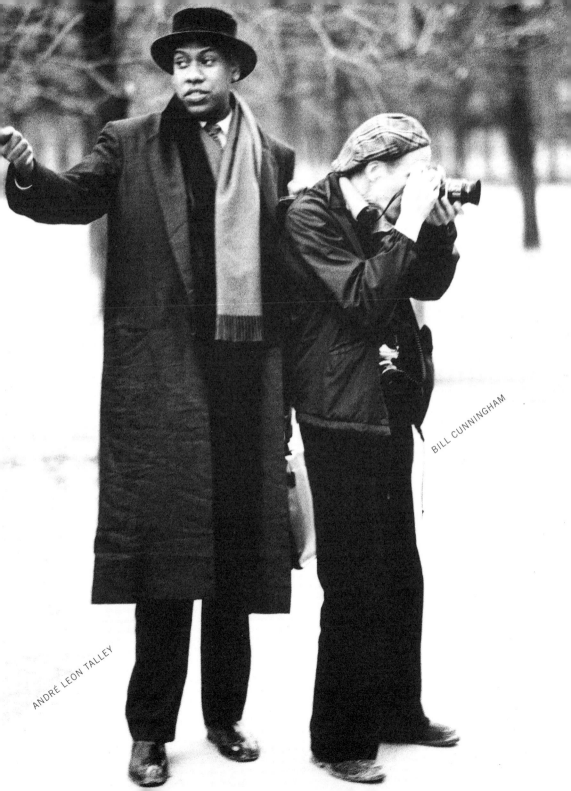

ANDRÉ LEON TALLEY

BILL CUNNINGHAM

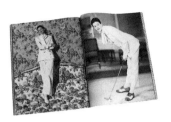

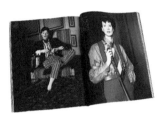

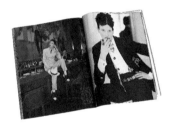

"I'M TWENTY-EIGHT, AND I'M ORIGINALLY FROM BUFFALO, NEW YORK. I STARTED MODELING TEN YEARS AGO AND WAS TOLD I WAS TOO OLD THEN. ■ MY LOOK ISN'T COMMERCIAL. MY SMILE IS CROOKED, I'M FIVE FOOT TEN WITH GIANT BONES AND BIG KNEES AND RED HAIR. I'M MANLY, IN A WAY. ■ I WASN'T A STAR—MY AGENTS WEREN'T CALLING ME. NO ONE WAS PAYING ATTENTION TO ME. I HAD NOTHING TO LOSE, SO I FELT I COULD BE MYSELF. I PLUCKED MY EYE-BROWS OUT DURING A SHOOT WITH STEVEN MEISEL. MY CONFIDENCE LEVEL WITH MY LOOKS SHOT UP. ■ I'VE NEVER HAD TO SLEEP WITH A PHOTOGRAPHER FOR A JOB."

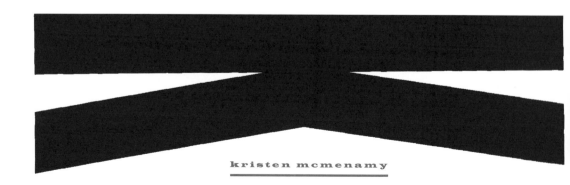

kristen mcmenamy

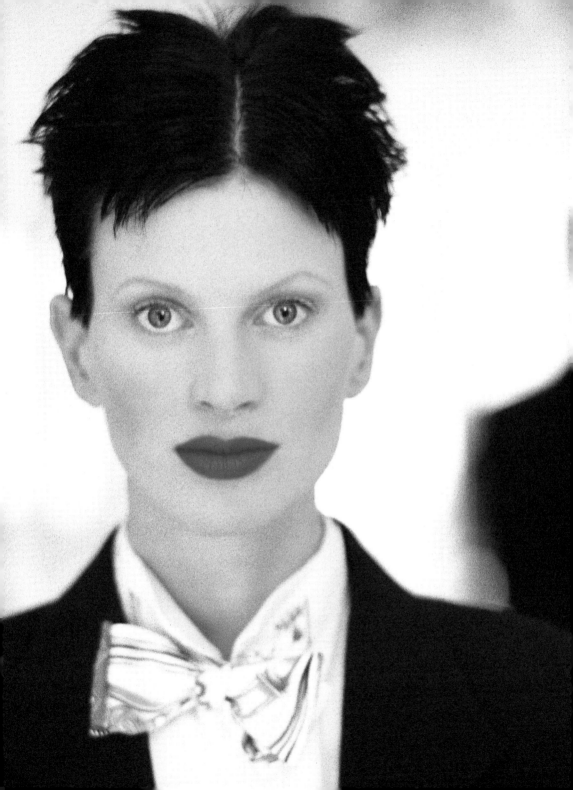

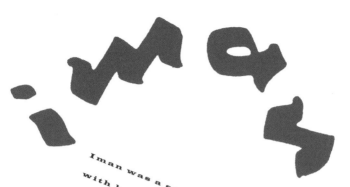

iman

Iman was a special commodity. The first time I worked with her, I was introduced to her at night. She was wearing white. I thought she was absolutely beautiful. She looked like what she was—an African princess.

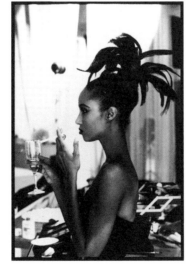

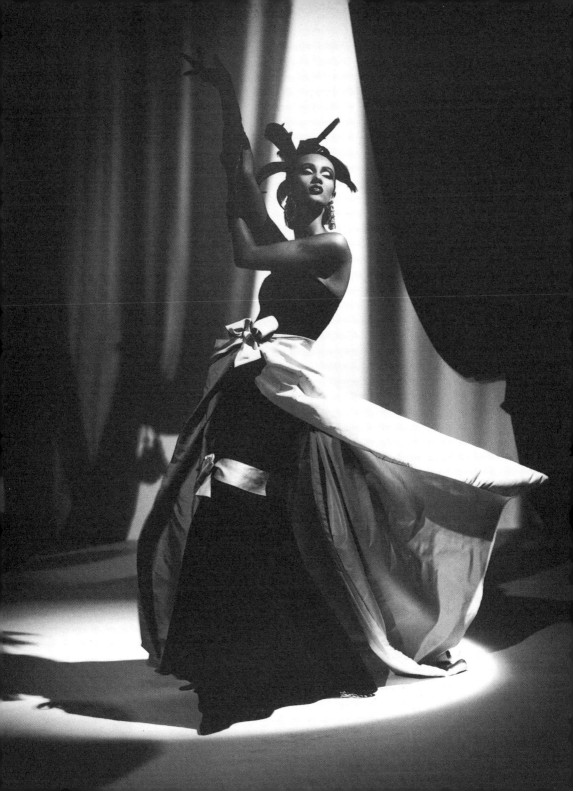

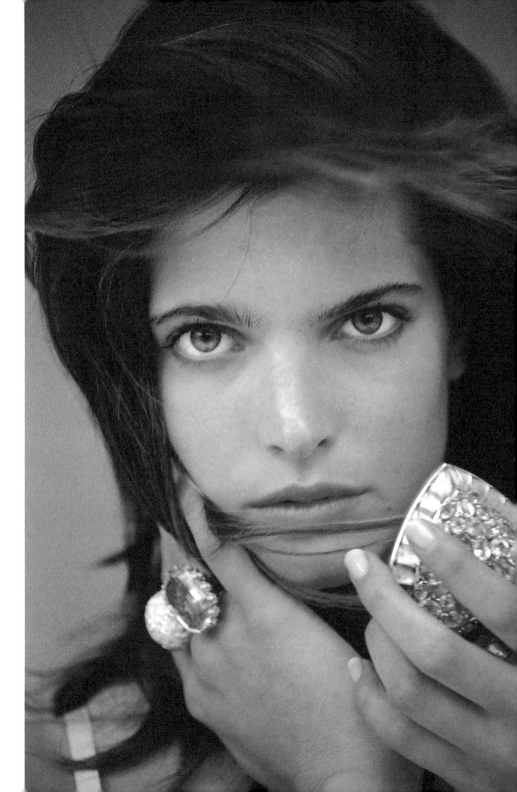

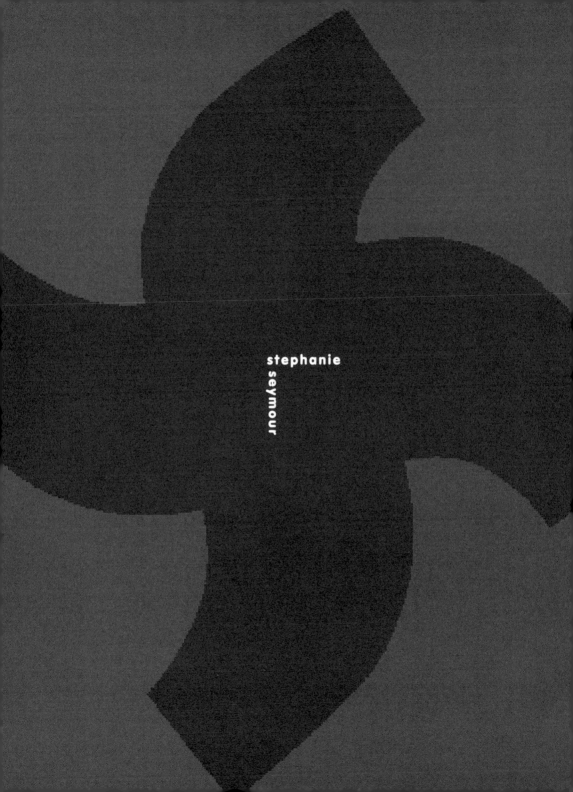

stephanie
seymour

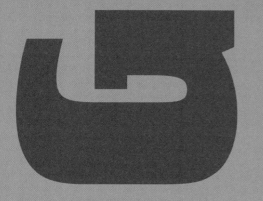

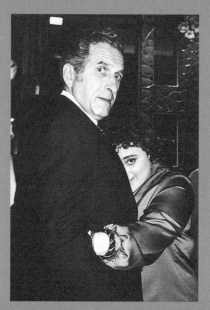

MONIQUE PILLARD

"IF YOU WANT TO BE A STAR, YOU'D

BETHANN HARDISON

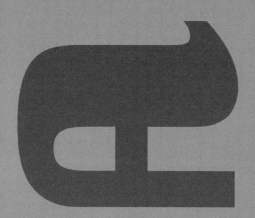

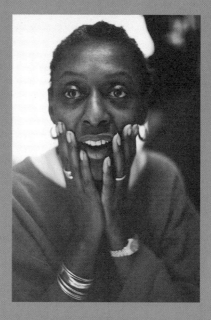

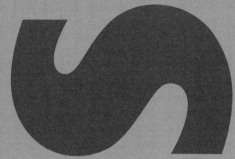

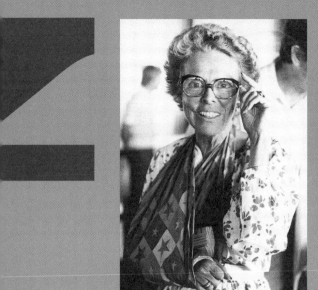

EILEEN FORD

BETTER BE PREPARED TO PAY FOR IT"
— BETHANN HARDISON

KAREN MULDER, GERALD MARIE

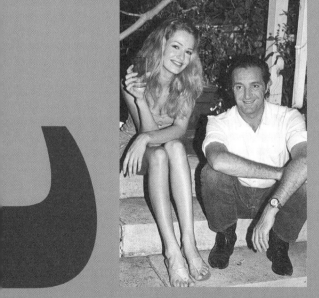

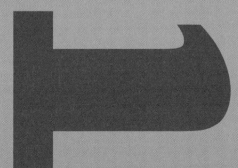

AGENTS can be mothers or aunts to a girl, or they can be like gurus or Svengalis. But no matter how beautiful or talented the girl is, she needs someone to take charge and chart her career. I always tell a girl, "The best agent is the one who likes you the most."

FRANCES GRILL *president,* Click ★ Agents are like parents—they give life to models, protect, nurture, give them direction, and help them realize their own value and power. They are so young, just out of school, and their lives have been completely controlled. We're here to support them and continue to give them direction. ★ I look for the small differences that expand on what is traditionally considered beautiful. Elle MacPherson, for example, had a mouth that most others considered too big. When I see a girl, I think about what it looks like behind the lens. The joy of this business is to trick the market a little. ★ I love to find girls raw, on the street or in the elevator. I found Whitney Houston in the lobby of Carnegie Hall, and Isabella Rossellini came to me through a mutual friend. She asked me if she could do something for me around the office and I said "Model." She was a good sport.

BETHANN HARDISON *president,* Bethann Management ★ You're always dealing with someone else's children. It helps to have a maternal mentality. I encourage the soul, I encourage the spirit, I encourage all the talents of a person. ★ Models are a special monster. A different species of athlete. They really want to win. ★ The first thing I look for is personality. She does have to be pretty, but talking with them tells me a lot. Personality, legs, skin, height—that can pull you through a lot of crap.

MONIQUE PILLARD *president,* Elite ★ **What do you look for in a model?** I like to take risks. You take a chance when you take in a Lucie de La Falaise. She's short, but she has attitude. Of the ones from the past, Bonnie Berman was exuberant—it was like sunshine just entered the room. It was a challenge to place Janice Dickenson. Same with Lauren Hutton, with the gap in her teeth. It's that *je ne sais quoi*. The attitude. Not just being beautiful.

Where do you find girls? I found one at a McDonald's in New Jersey. Carol Alt came into our office first because we were closest to the subway. ★ **Is it hard turning a girl away?** We live in the business of rejection. Only one is going to get the job. We try to help them build confidence. Girls are always coming up to me and saying, "Please give me a hug." ★ **What's your role in the model's life?** I teach them the fundamentals—you might teach the boxer how to duck a punch, but the technique is his own. You have to bring your own style into it. What I offer aren't promises but concrete propositions of work.

EILEEN FORD *cochairman with Jerry Ford,* Ford Models ★ **What does it take to be a top model?** A girl doesn't have to be beautiful in the classic sense of the word. Of course, if she wants to make any money, it helps. But more important, she has to have something inside herself that makes her come alive. It's an inner drive—I call it the X factor. It's the one thing I cannot control. ★ **How do you make a girl a success?** It's a matter of right time, right place. The photographer is everything. It's up to the model to make the photographer's vision come true. She's the chameleon. Models are creative in response to the creative desires of others. It might not happen with that first photo either. I've been watching a girl emerge—it's been one year since I took her in. She'd never even been to an art gallery. The trick is to graduate from a youngster to a star. ★ **How long does a girl live with you?** It might be as little as one week. Jerry Hall lived with me for about a year. We did yoga every morning at 7 A.M. ★ **Out of the 10,000 letters you receive a year and 7,000 visits, how many models actually make it to that stage?** After working with about forty, I find that four or five really good ones emerge. ★ **Is it hard to reject a girl?** It's the nicest thing I can do for a girl who isn't pretty enough to be a model. She has to get on with her life.

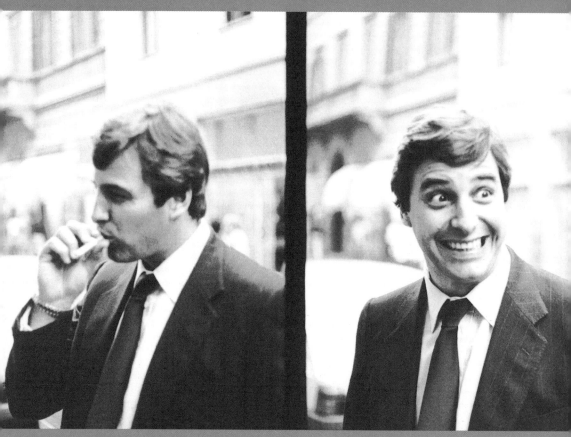

JOHN CASABLANCAS

- -

CINDY CRAWFORD: I have dinner all the time with my agents, but we're not best friends. If I need to make a decision that's hard or if I have to say something that's unpleasant, I have the freedom to do that without damaging a friendship.

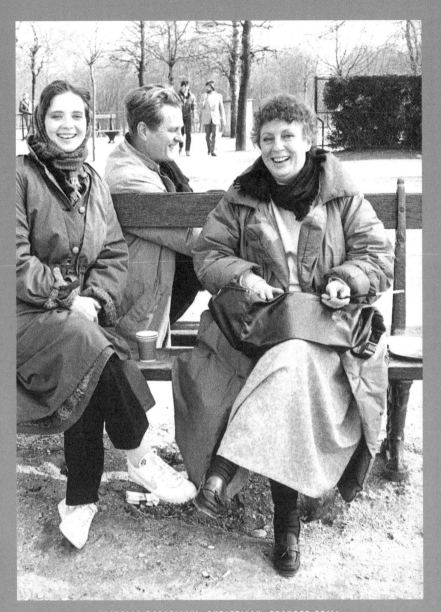

ISABELLA ROSSELLINI, CHRISTIAAN, FRANCES GRILL

LINDA EVANGELISTA: You can't do it without an agent. You can't do it on your own. You have to shop and shop until you find the right one.

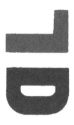

louise despointes

"what's important in this business is giving the public a dream they can relate to."

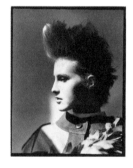

juliette

"I STARTED MY OWN AGENCY, CITY MODELS, IN PARIS IN 1979. I STARTED A SISTER AGENCY, CALLED NAME, IN NEW YORK IN 1984 . I HAD BEEN A MODEL IN THE LATE SIXTIES, AND AT THAT TIME THE FASHION WORLD WAS QUITE DIFFERENT THAN IT IS NOW—LESS COMMERCIAL, MORE CREATIVE. ● I WANTED TO FIND A NEW BREED OF MODELS WHO WERE DIFFERENT, MORE REAL-LOOKING, NOT THOSE GLOSSY GIRLS WHO WERE SUCH A PART OF THE INDUSTRY AT THE TIME. ● THE MODEL-AGENT RELATIONSHIP IS A LITTLE LIKE WHAT HAPPENS WHEN TWO PEOPLE FALL IN LOVE: THEY'RE BOTH LOOKING FOR RESPECT, SPIRIT, PERSONALITY AND BEAUTY. MORE THAN ANYTHING ELSE, WHAT MAKES A GREAT MODEL IS INTELLIGENCE."

LOUISE DESPOINTES HAD AN EYE FOR A CERTAIN KIND OF GIRL. SHE WAS VERY GOOD AT TUNING INTO THE TIME. THE MODELS SHE DISCOVERED—CECILIA CHANCELLOR, LESLIE WINER, JULIETTE AND LAETITIA FIRMIN DIDOT—BECAME THE INTELLIGENT ICONS OF THE INDUSTRY. CITY AND NAME WERE PRECURSORS TO THE SMALLER AGENCIES OF TODAY.

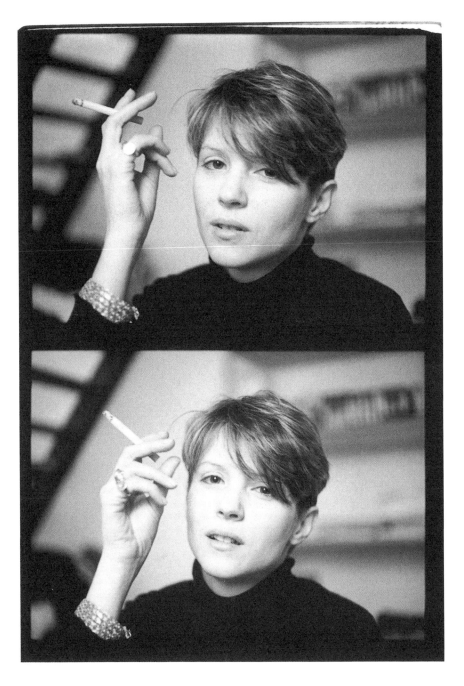

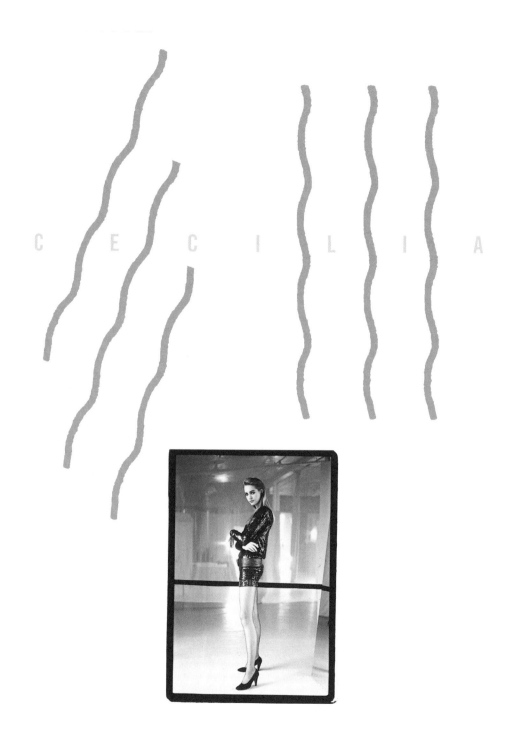

CECILIA

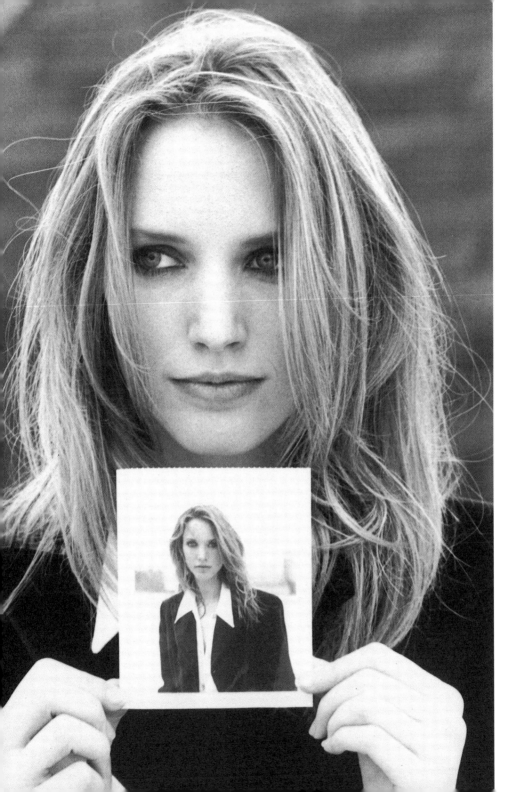

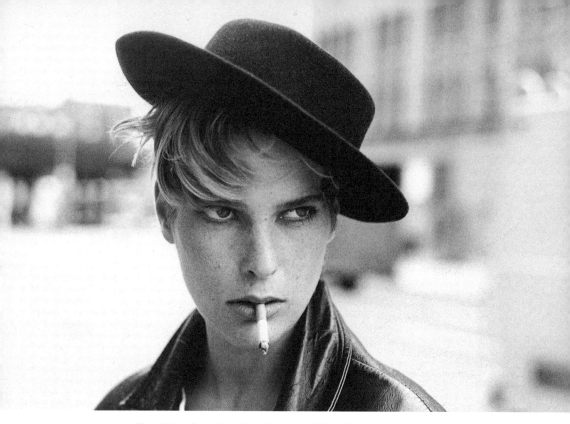

LESLIE WINER

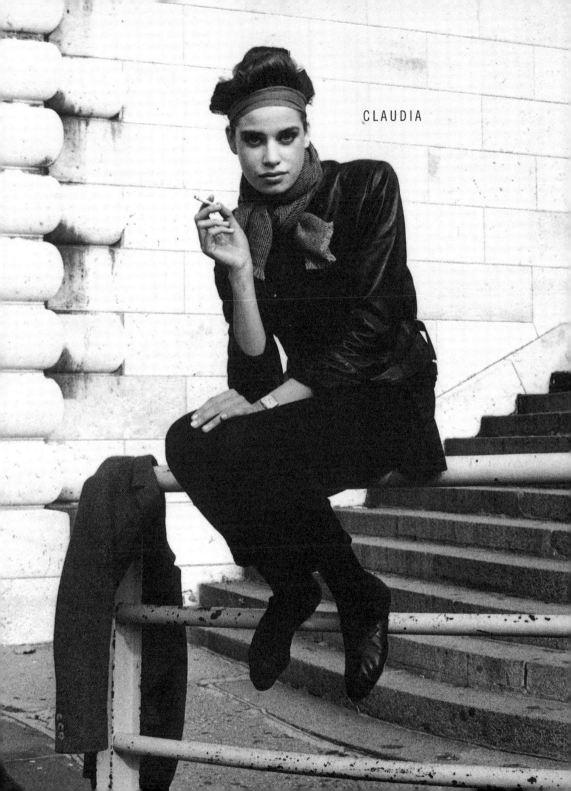

CLAUDIA

"I ALWAYS HATED TO SAY I WAS A
MODEL. I NEVER CHANGED THE COLOR
OF MY HAIR. I BITE MY NAILS. I WAS
SHY AND I HATED TO MOVE IN FRONT
OF THE CAMERA, BUT THE BEST
THING IS I MET THE MAN OF MY LIFE
DOING THIS JOB."

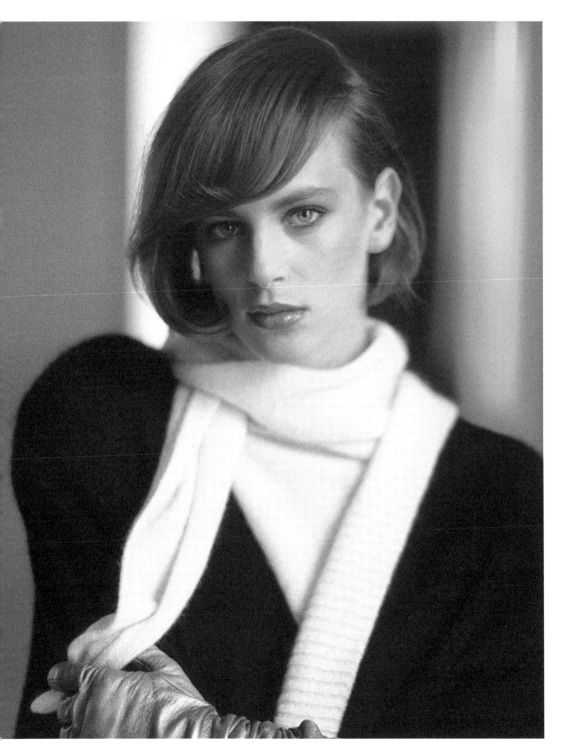

LAETITIA FIRMIN DIDOT

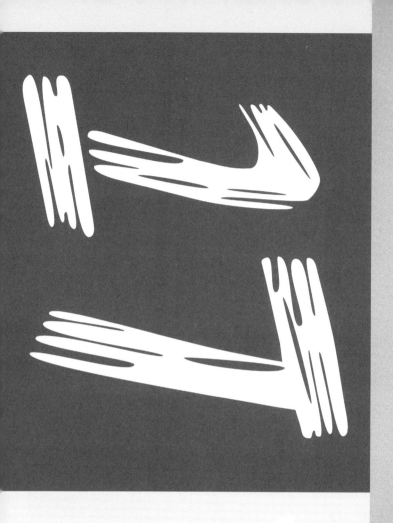

LISA TAYLOR

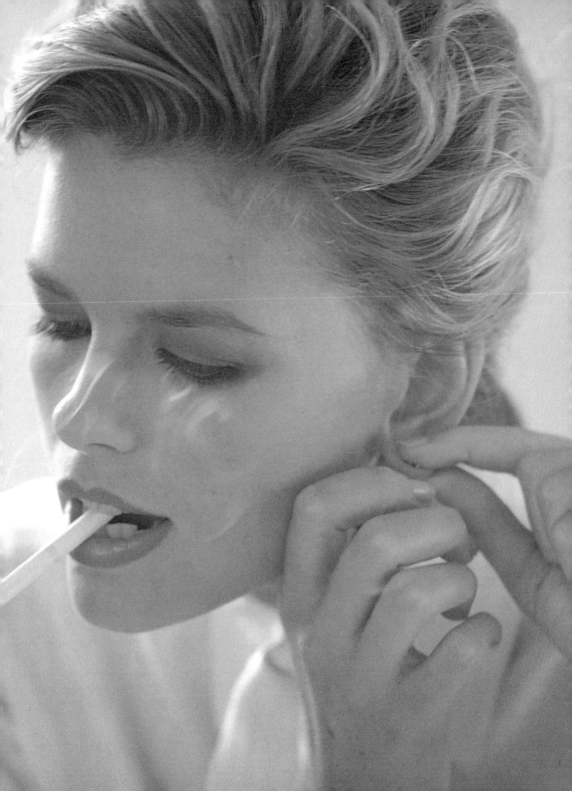

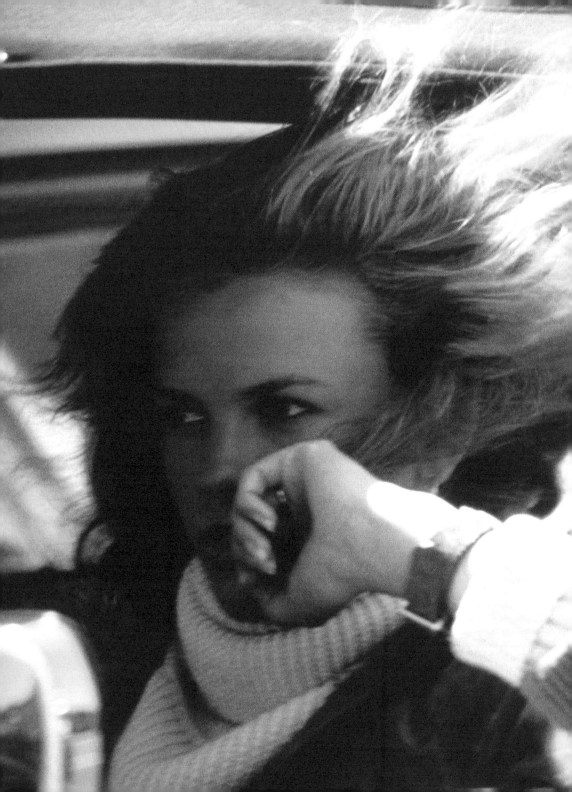

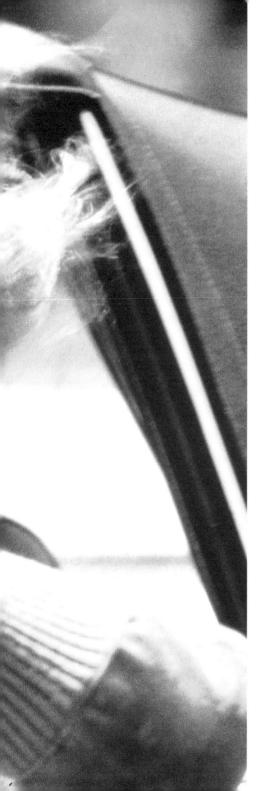

When I first met

Lisa Taylor...

...she looked like a sporty rich kid. On our very first go-see, she carried my tripod. I photographed her wearing a peasant dress and black tights. She was quite beautiful, but the early pictures seemed pretty static until the day we sat her in a Mercedes 450SL for

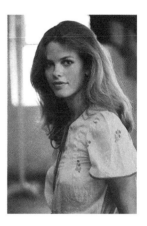

American *Vogue*. It was Polly Mellen's idea. We were so unsophisticated back then. We didn't even have a walkie-talkie. I was in a van next to her with a zoom lens, shouting directions, and Christiaan had squeezed down into the jump seat with his combs and brushes. We just went back and forth over the George Washington Bridge until somebody eventually told us to stop. This was 1975, and even today the shot reflects a certain timeless quality—the modern woman who has something on her mind and is going places fast.

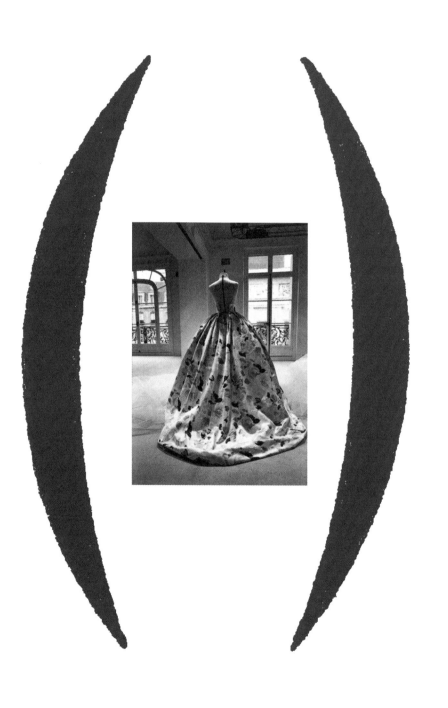

DESIGNERS

THE REASON WE'RE ALL IN THIS BUSINESS IS BECAUSE OF THE CLOTHES. IT ALL STARTS IN EUROPE WITH THE FABRIC HOUSES, BUT IT'S THE DESIGNERS WHO MAKE IT ALL GLAMOROUS. IN THE PAST FIF-TEEN YEARS, DESIGNERS HAVE ALSO HAD AN ENORMOUS INFLUENCE ON MODELS' CAREERS BY USING MAGAZINE GIRLS INSTEAD OF HOUSE MODELS TO SHOW THEIR DESIGNS ON THE RUNWAY. IT'S THE DESIGNER NOW WHO CAN MAKE A MODEL A LEGEND.

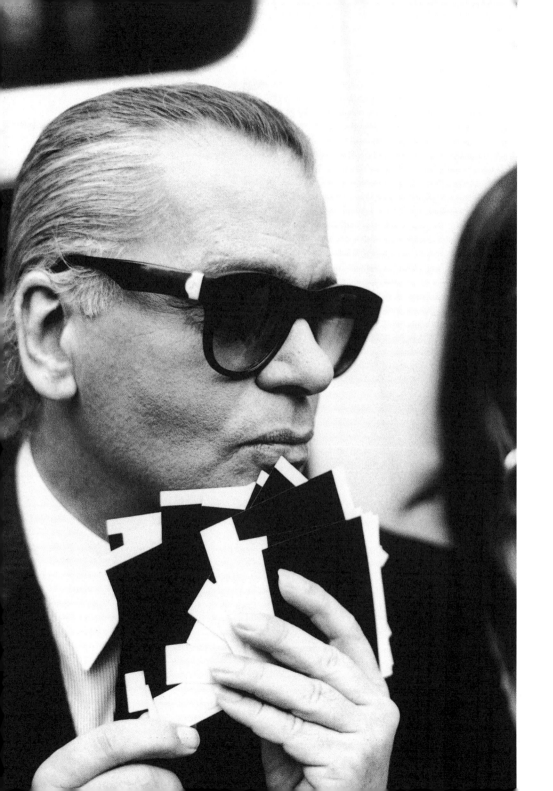

karl lagerfeld

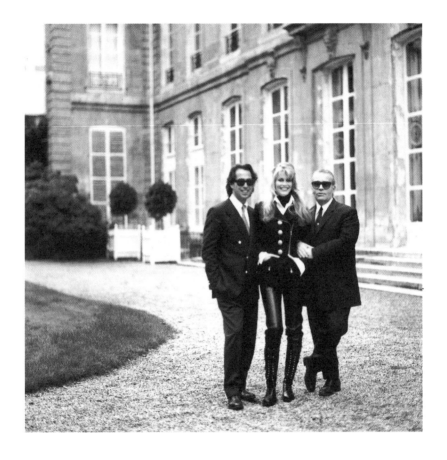

KARL IS THE QUINTESSENTIAL EUROPEAN DESIGNER. HE HAS THE ABILITY TO DO IT
ALL AND NOT LOOK SHOOK UP ABOUT IT. HE ALWAYS ENJOYS HIMSELF, AND THAT
COMES THROUGH IN EVERYTHING HE DOES. KARL'S MUSES OF THE MOMENT:
CLAUDIA SCHIFFER AND KRISTEN MCMENAMY.

GRÈS
COUTURE

THIS IS WHERE IT ALL CAME FROM, IN SALONS LIKE THOSE OF THE LATE MADAME GRÈS, WHERE THERE IS NOT A SOUND TO BE HEARD BUT THE RUSTLING OF TAFFETA. NO MUSIC. NO SUPERSTAR MODELS. THE DAY I SHOT THESE PHOTOS, I WAS SO EXCITED—I HAPPENED TO BE WALKING IN JUST WHEN CECIL BEATON ARRIVED.

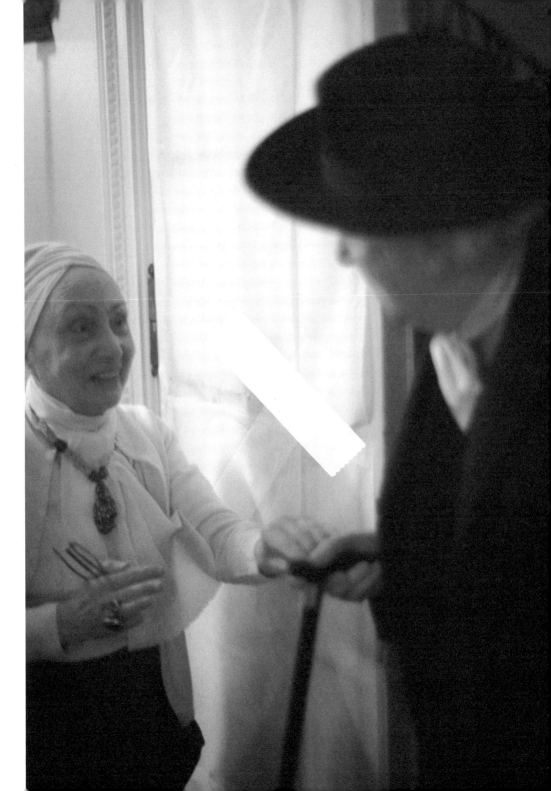

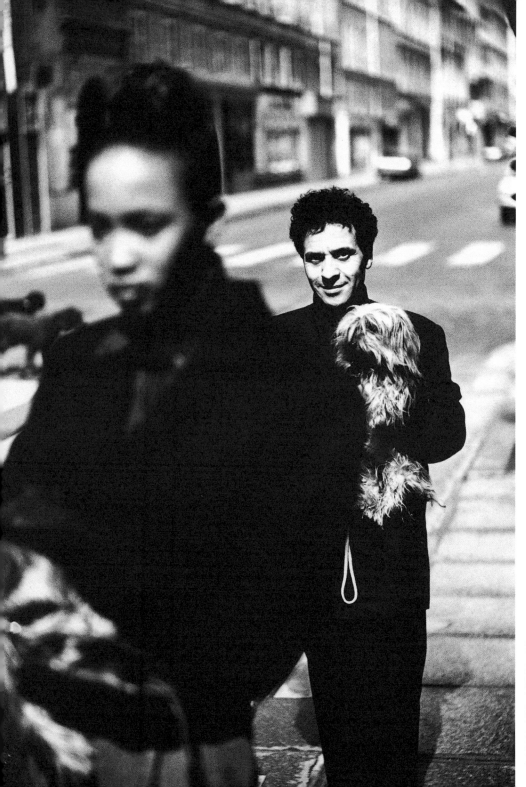

azzedine alaïa

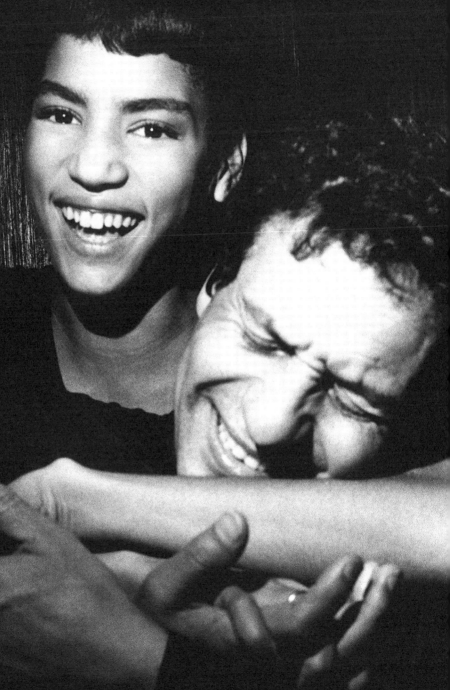

WHEN I FIRST MET AZZEDINE IN PARIS, HE WAS PINNING AND SEWING AWAY AND CUTTING PATTERNS. THERE WERE ONLY FOUR PEOPLE AT THE TIME, THERE MAY STILL BE— IT'S A FAMILY BUSINESS, WHERE THEY ALL DO EVERYTHING FROM IRONING TO CLEANING UP. AZZEDINE HAS A QUIET TUNISIAN CHARM AND IS THE ONLY ONE I SPEAK MY BROKEN FRENCH TO.

HE'S VERY GENEROUS AND ALL THE MODELS LOVE HIM.

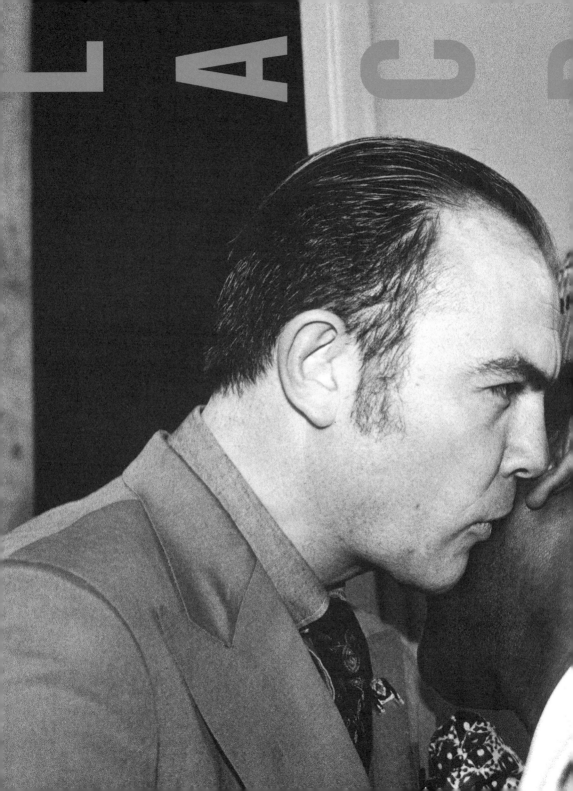

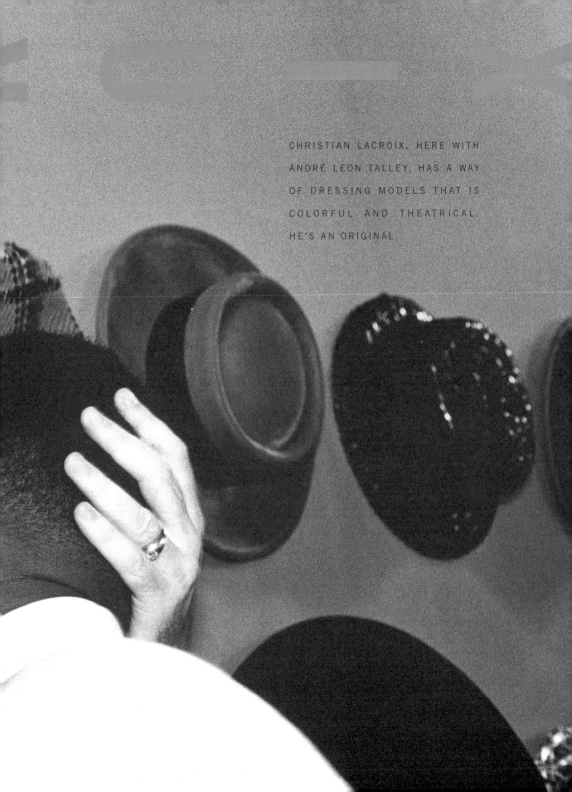

CHRISTIAN LACROIX, HERE WITH
ANDRÉ LEON TALLEY, HAS A WAY
OF DRESSING MODELS THAT IS
COLORFUL AND THEATRICAL.
HE'S AN ORIGINAL.

yves saint laurent

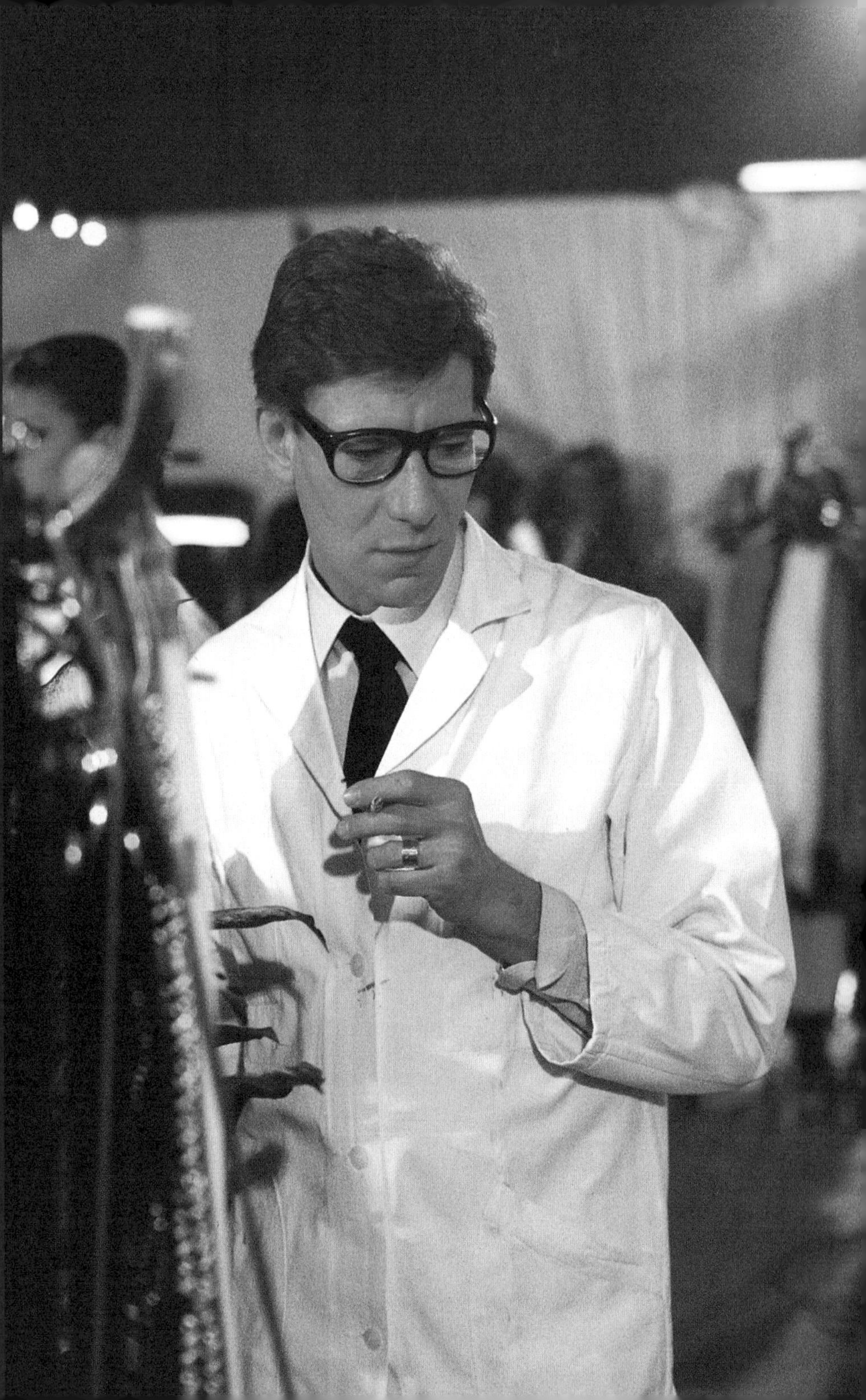

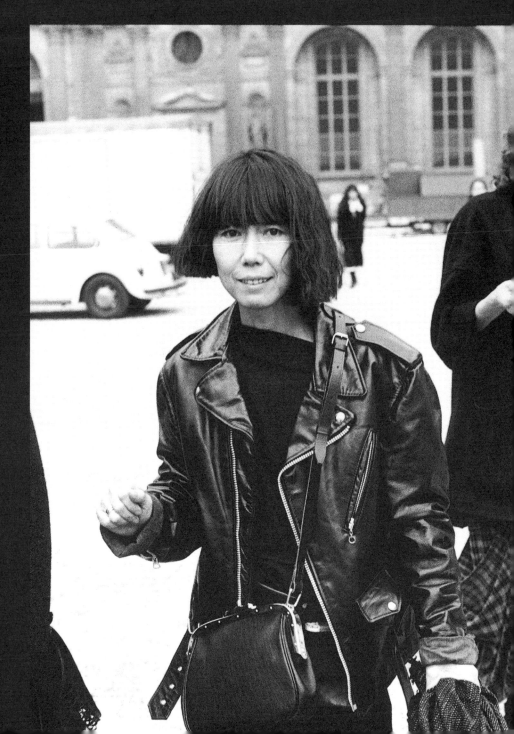

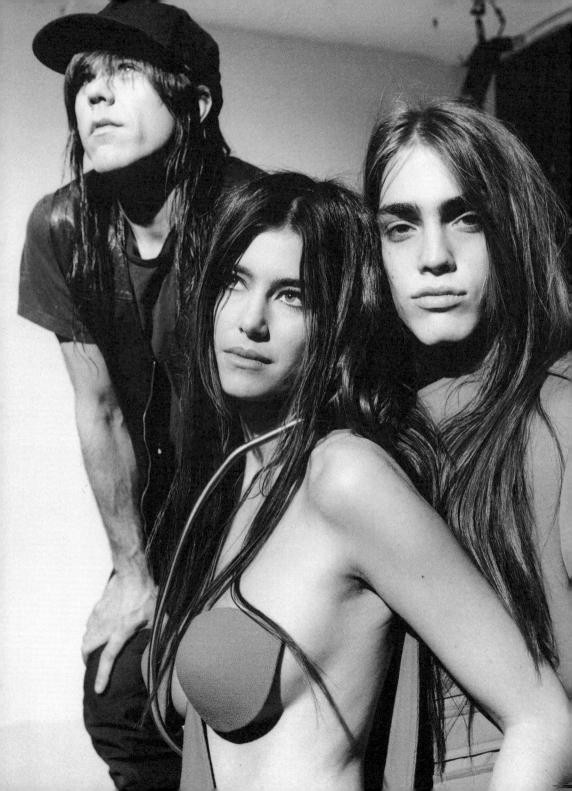

marc jacobs

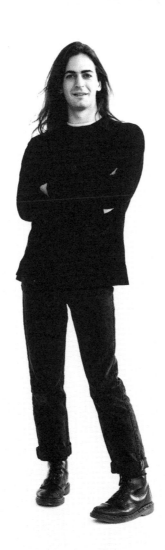

"I LIKE DOING RUNWAY WORK, BECAUSE IT'S SPONTANEOUS AND LIVE. WHATEVER HAPPENS, HAPPENS—YOU JUST HAVE TO GO WITH IT. WHEN I'M DOING THE RUNWAY, I TAKE THE VIBES OFF THE AUDIENCE. I CAN TELL IN THE FIRST FIVE MINUTES WHEN EVERYBODY LOVES IT. I JUST FEEL ELECTRIC!"

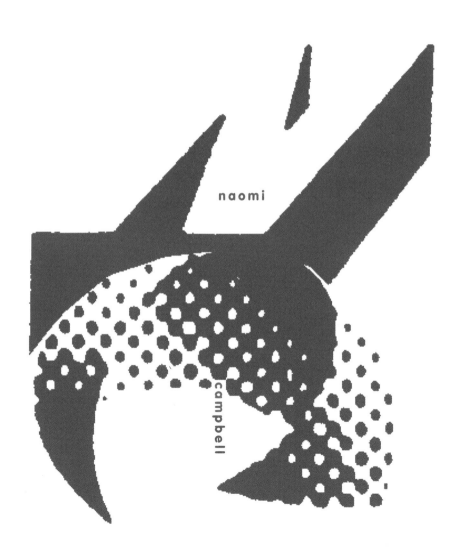

naomi

campbell

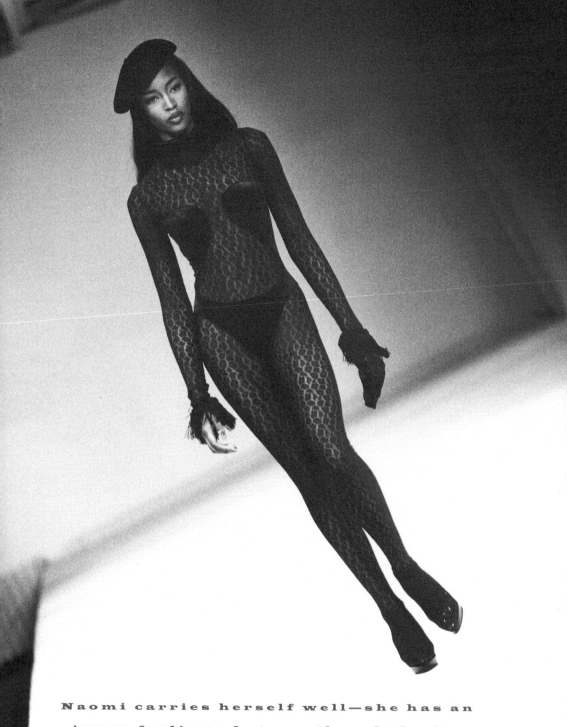

Naomi carries herself well—she has an
inner feeling of strength and clarity

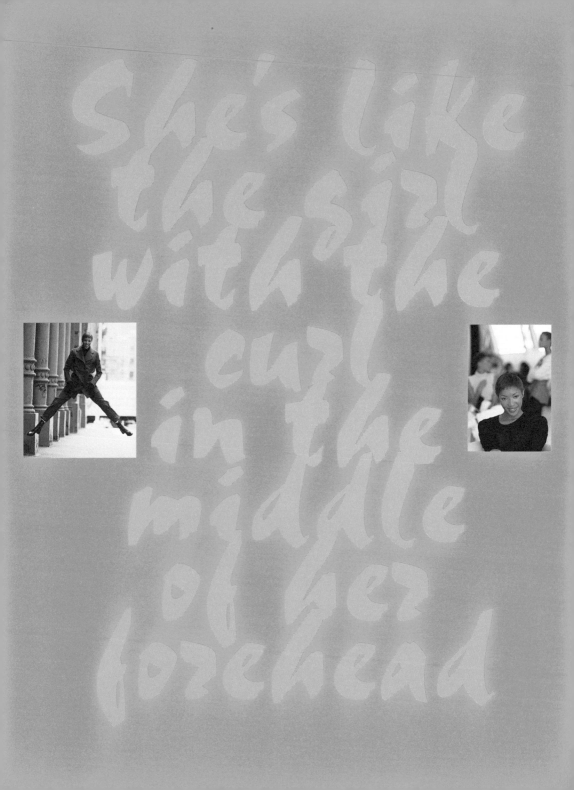

She's like the girl with the curl in the middle of her forehead

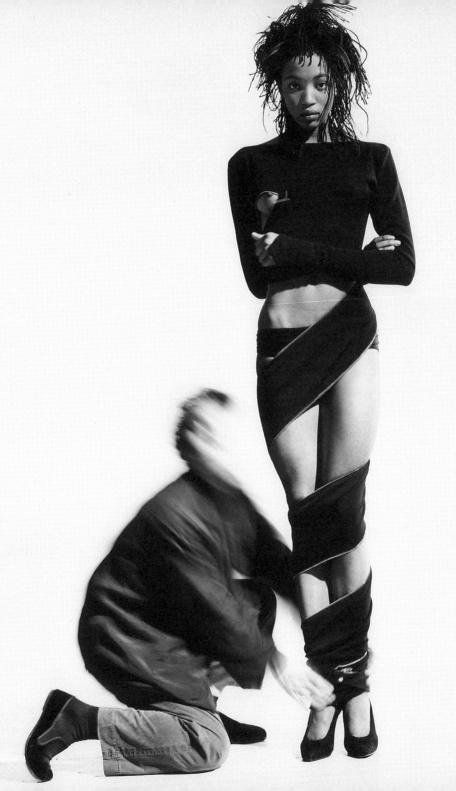

"Twenty years from now, I see myself with my children in a house with my husband in front of the fireplace and me cooking dinner."

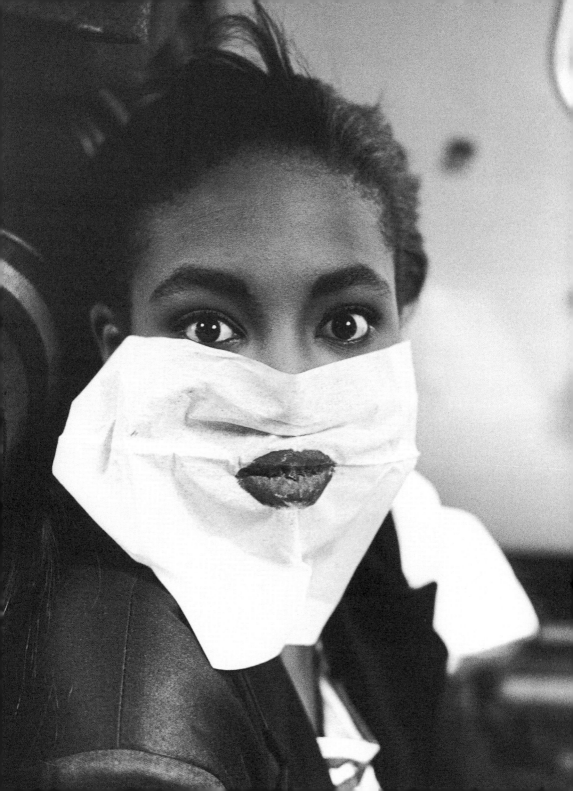

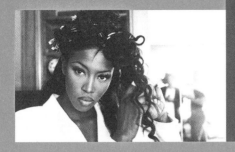

"If you're going to get into this business, stay balanced and in contact with your family. Soon as something happens, Mum is the first one I call. She danced, so it's kind of the same thing...she was the only black girl in her group in Geneva. She used to have people steal from her and rip up her costumes. My mum warned me to be careful."

"When you're in front of the camera, you always have to remember that you're modeling clothes. So I have to look good in the outfit that I'm wearing. It's a collaboration between the photographer and the hair and makeup people. I'm the end result of their work. It's much better when you feel something from the photographer—otherwise the picture comes out and I look lost."

"The reward of advertising work rarely comes to blacks. I feel taken advantage of in certain ways, but I look at this as something I'm doing for black people in general."

"When I first started out in this business, I used to get really depressed if I was rejected. But my mother told me, 'You can't take it personally.' She's right. You are looked at as a number, in a way."

"The way to get covers sometimes is to ask for them. I asked for my first *Vogue* cover, the French one. I didn't used to but I saw Linda Evangelista asking for hers."

"Since I was three years old, I've been dancing. Now that I'm into modeling, I just can't let it go. Now I'm dancing and singing too. We'll see how it goes. It's not like taking a picture and you're done at the end of the day. It goes on and on. I just want to try a new career. It may not work, but at least I can say that I tried."

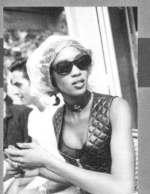

"My most embarrassing moment was on the runway. My pants, my skirt, everything came down. It was at the fourth show. I just pulled it all up and went on walking."

"I don't always wear underwear. When I'm in the heat especially, I can't wear it. Like, if I'm wearing a flowing dress, why do I have to wear underwear?"

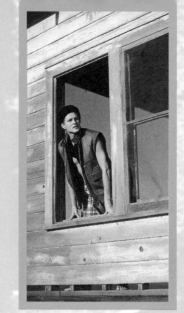
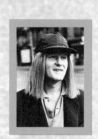
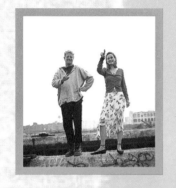
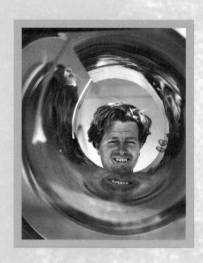
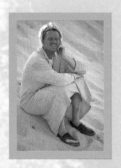

CHRIS

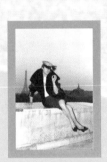

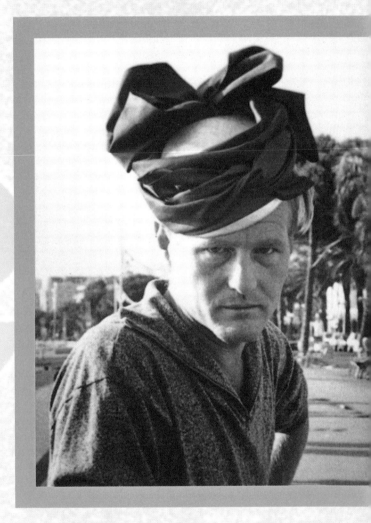

TIAAN

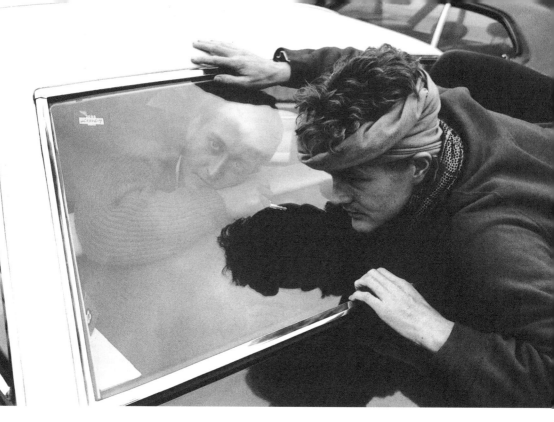

"i like style—real style. it comes down to the heart."

How did you get into this business? I left my father's barbershop in a small Dutch village and by a lucky fluke ended up creative director in New York for Bergdorf Goodman's beauty salon. That was 1967. It included going to photographers' studios and fashion shows to take care of models' hair on the spot. It was a new concept, because until that time models would simply go to the salon, get the coif nailed down and then go to work. From there, I stumbled into the most enviable job in the world. **What was the modeling world like back then?** When I started, there was Twiggy, Penelope Tree, Verushka. Then it became the domain of a group of well-bred moneyed girls who kind of sported modeling, like Elsa Peretti and Marina Schiano. Then followed the girls who became professional models—Rosie Vela, Patti Hansen, Lisa Taylor. That's when I first noticed that the chosen girls were like adopted kids to the powers that ruled. Girls they would have wanted as daughters. Then nature took over in the mid-Seventies, early Eighties, with Lisa Ryall and Kim Alexis. Soul became a must. From there, the recent surge to glamour. **From your perspective, who creates the supermodel?** I learned that no matter what your eye sees and thinks about anyone, it remains the photographers' exclusive domain to get excited about who transfers to film best. There is the mystery.

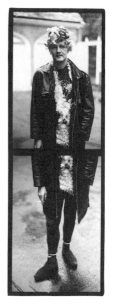

"beauty is how you treat people and treat yourself."

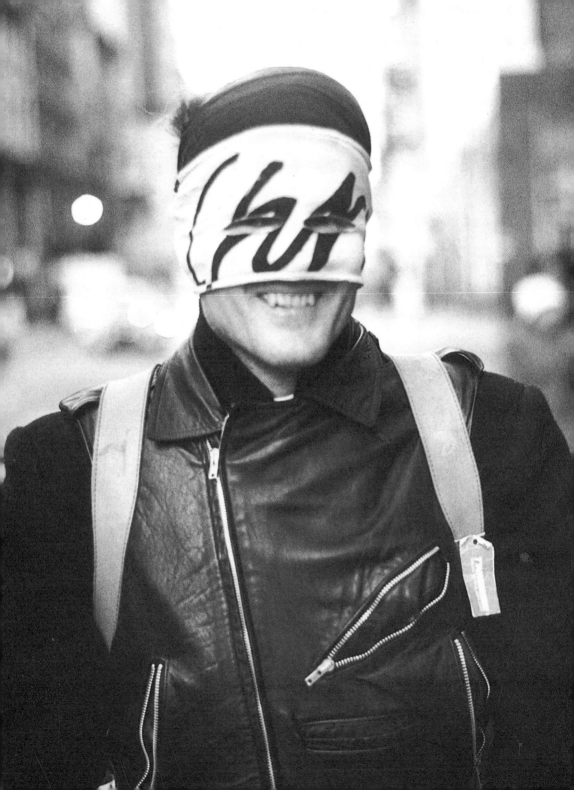

Christiaan is a genius at easing models into the middle of the set, and then he just does the hair there. He's the ultimate catalyst, the first one to get hold of the girl that day and set the mood.

What is involved in doing hair for photography? You have to know how to do good hair and you have to have some extra sensory perception. To do good hair, you've got to feel the pulse of the whole thing – and see the hair relating to the clothes. Hair gives the sense of the woman and the clothes are just put on. **How do you do what you do?** I start by saying hello to the hair with my hands, chat with the girl and I try to create an image that pleases. **How do you see your role?** The model and the photographer are often strangers. They find each other in generally embarrassing circumstances. I function as a friendly foil. **What is your technique to get them together creatively?** My being an extrovert allows girls to be more open themselves. If you clown around a bit, it makes it easier for them. It's a touch and feel job that sets up the girl's senses. Extremely delicate work. If you hit the mark, she blooms; If you miss, she wilts. **What does it take to be a top model?** There isn't any grand scheme in this business. You could hardly plan your way to become a top model, It is a chain of events. **What about the glamour side of the business?** I don't trust it. It makes me think of subjugating people. I'm always a little suspicious of glamorous people. What you see may not be what you get!

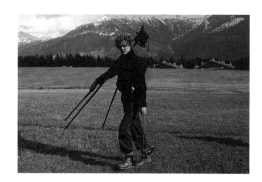

"THE PHONE RINGS AND YOU ARE ON YOUR WAY TO ARUBA, THEN BALI, THEN CAIRO. NO TIME FOR LAUNDRY AND DIRTY DISHES LEFT IN THE SINK. PRACTICALLY LIVING A DOUBLE LIFE. STILL, WHAT A WAY TO BE A TEENAGER...."

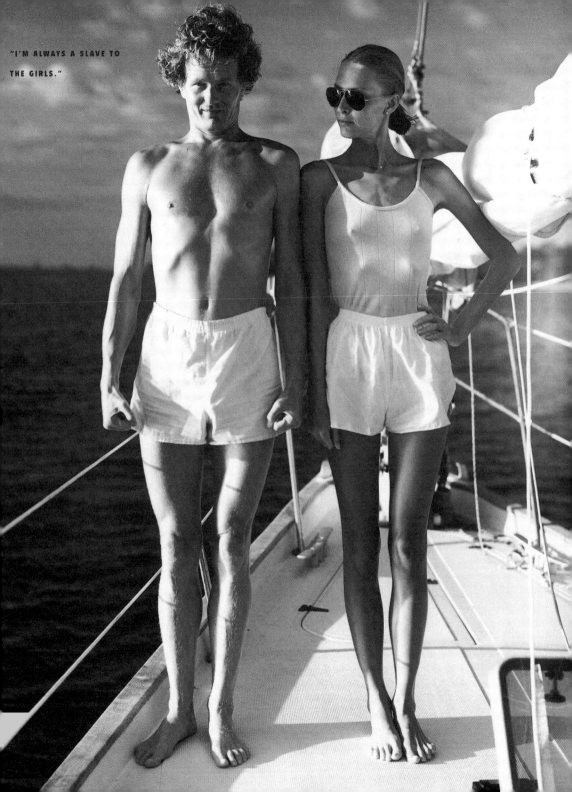

"I'M ALWAYS A SLAVE TO
THE GIRLS."

"ONCE, WE WERE AT THE COUTURE SHOWS IN ROME. I WAS DOING A *WEST SIDE STORY* THING ON TOP OF THE SPANISH STEPS. I JUMPED AND FELL AND SHATTERED MY HEEL. IT'S ONE OF THE HAZARDS OF THE JOB. I DID EVERYONE'S HAIR FROM MY BEDSIDE."

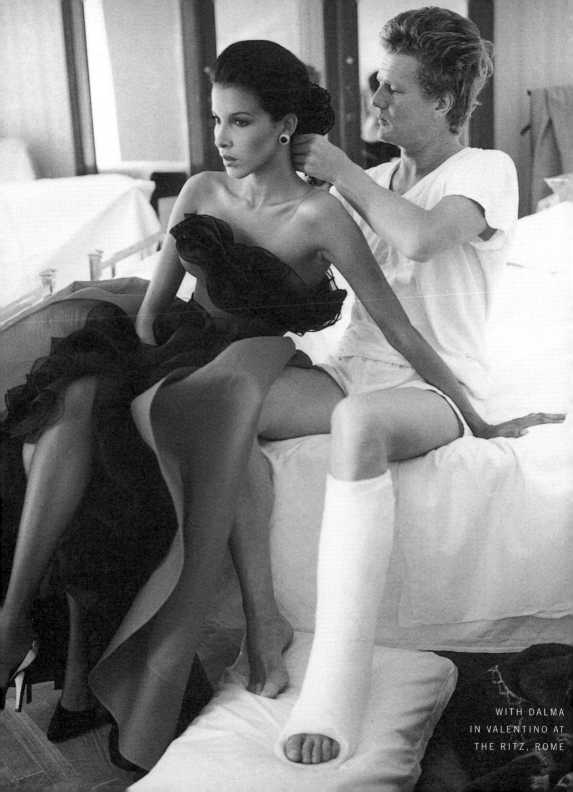

WITH DALMA
IN VALENTINO AT
THE RITZ, ROME

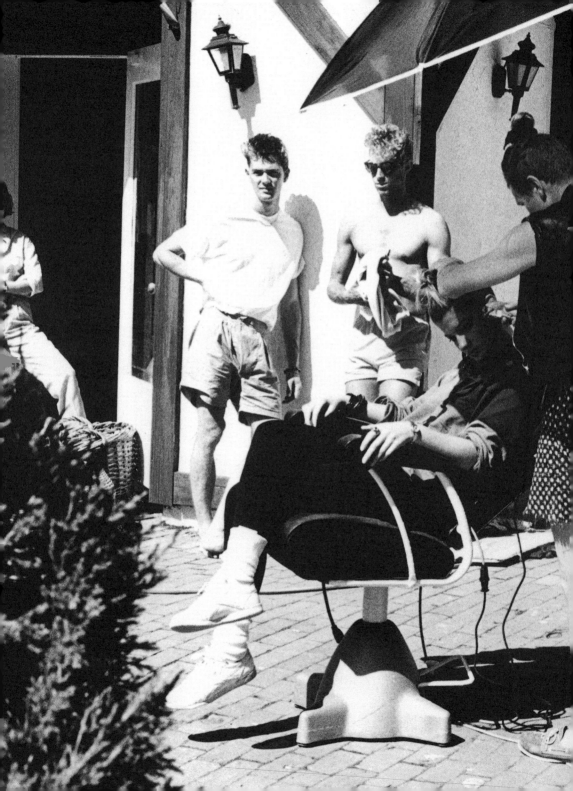

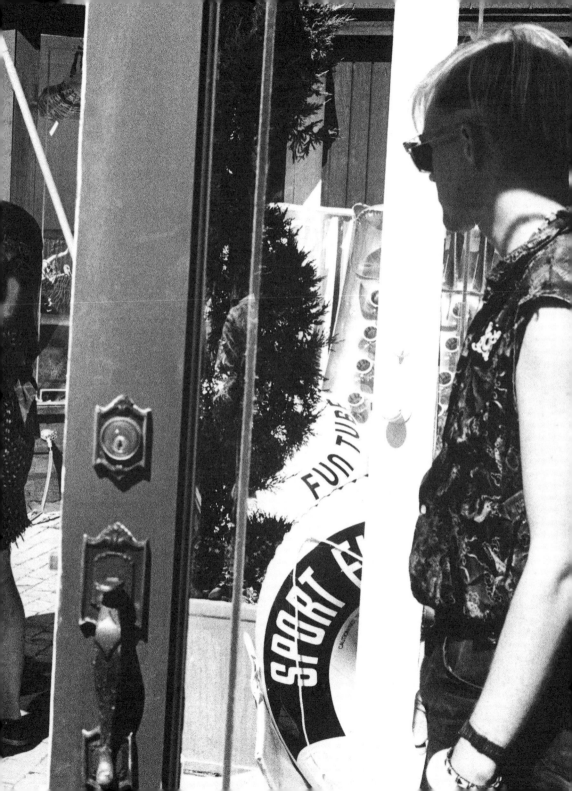

"MODELS ARE AN ENVIABLE BUNCH.

THEY'RE LIFTED OUT OF THE PACK AT

A TENDER AGE AND SENT OFF TO BE

WOOED, WINED AND DINED. THEN, IF

IT STICKS, THEY GO ON TO FAME AND

FORTUNE BEFORE THEY ARE ELIGIBLE

FOR THEIR DRIVER'S LICENSE."

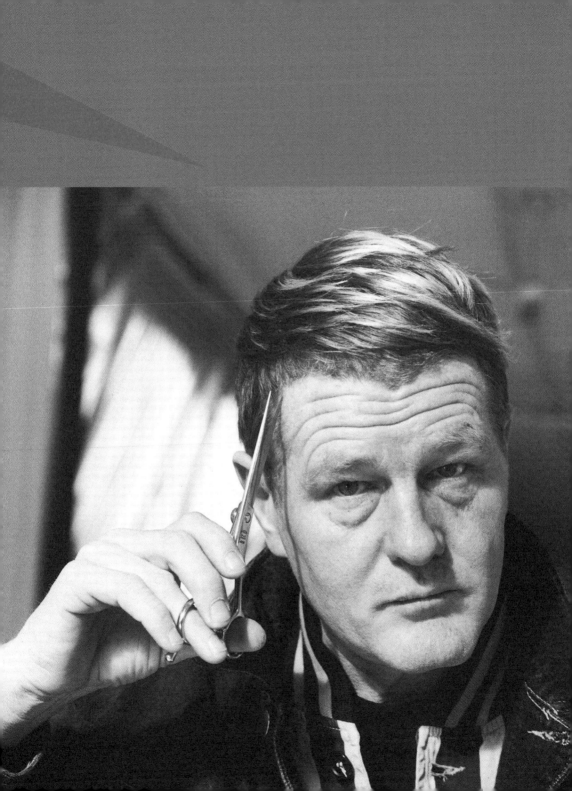

BETWEEN 1969 AND THE EARLY EIGHTIES, I PHOTOGRAPHED HUNDREDS OF MODELS. THE

REALLY GOOD ONES HAVE SUPPLIED ME WITH INSPIRATION. I CAN REMEMBER QUITE CLEARLY

THE DAY EACH OF THESE PICTURES WERE TAKEN. MOST ARE STOLEN SHOTS OF GIRLS WHO

HAVE JUST WALKED IN THE DOOR OF MY STUDIO WITHOUT HAVING HAD THEIR HAIR AND

MAKEUP DONE OR THEY CAPTURE A MOMENT WHEN THE MODEL IS LOOKING NATURAL AND

RELAXED BEFORE OR AFTER A DAY'S WORK. THIS IS A LOOK BACK AT GREAT EXAMPLES OF

THE MEMORABLE MODELS WHO ARE A MAJOR PART OF MY BIG PICTURE.

RECENT
PAST

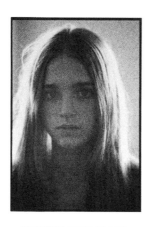

BONNIE'S FIRST GO-SEE

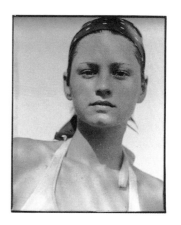

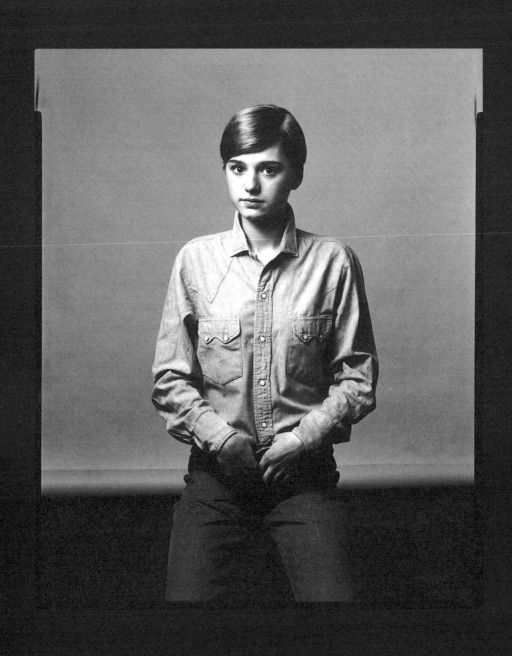

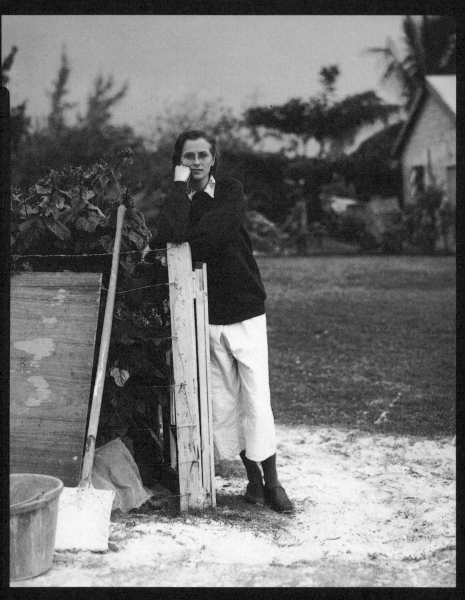

BONNIE PFEIFER, 1975

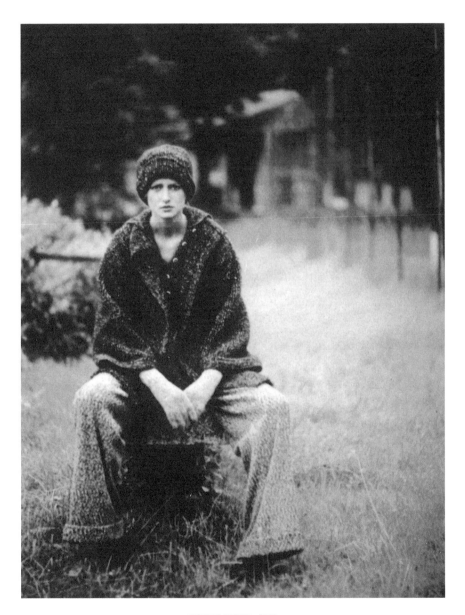

SHELLY SMITH, 1971

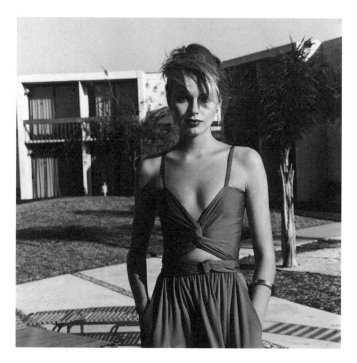

KIM CHARLTON, 1977

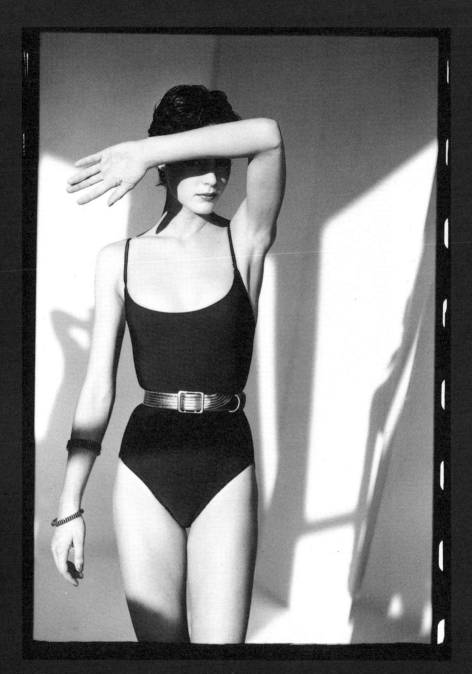

ESMÉ, 1979

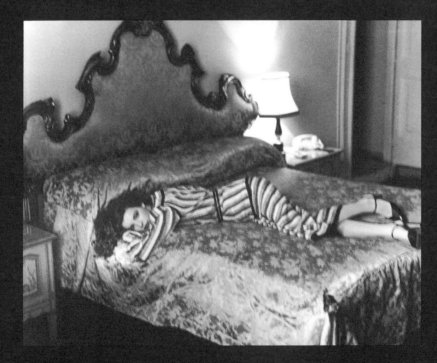

PRUDENCE, ROMA, 1978

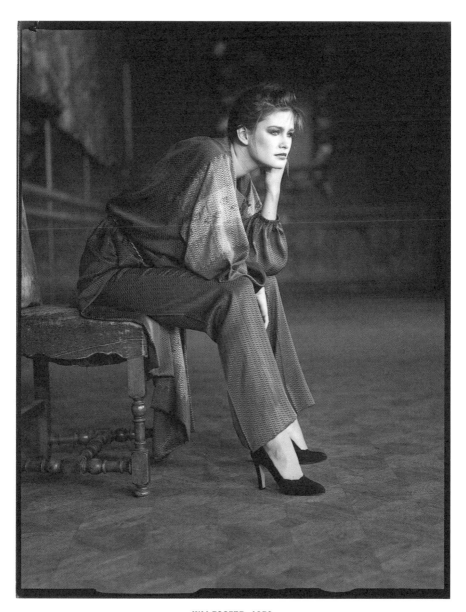

JULI FOSTER, 1978

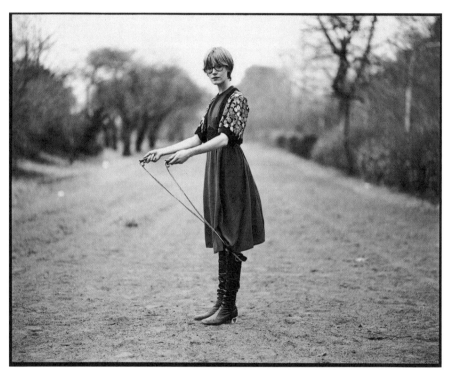

SUSAN MONCUR, TEST SHOT, CIRCA 1970

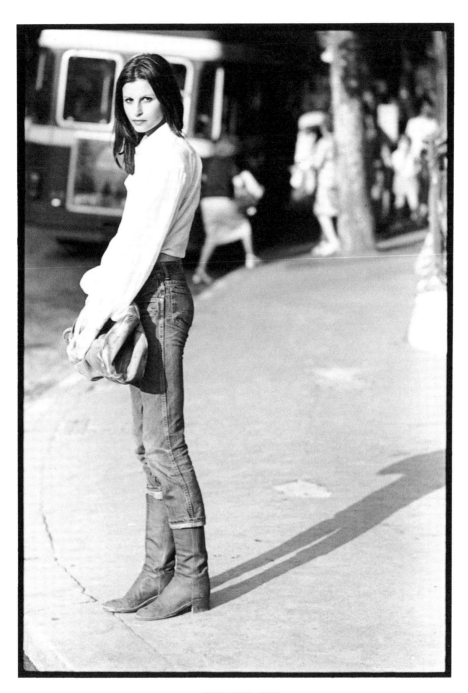

APOLLONIA, 1970

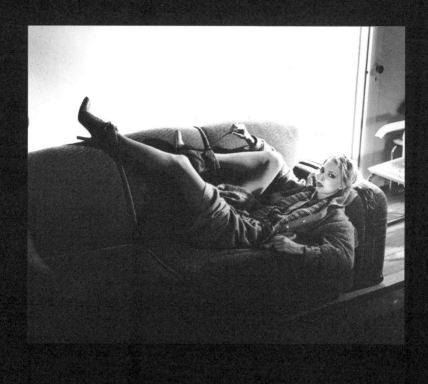
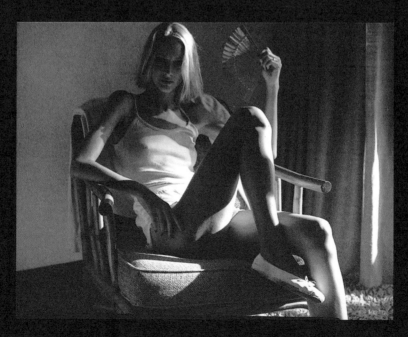

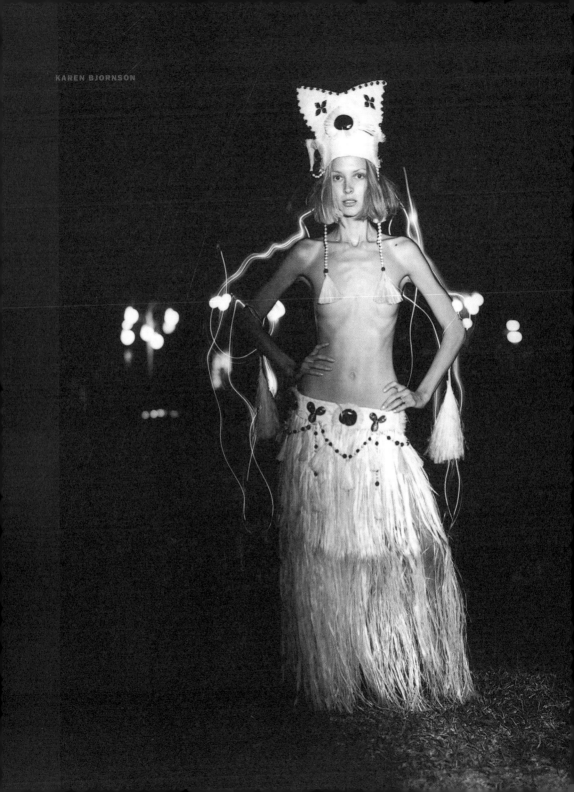

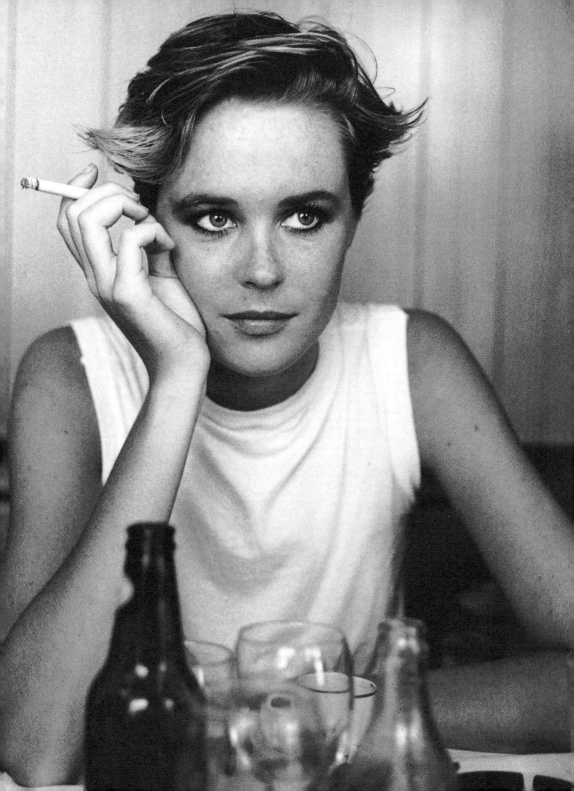

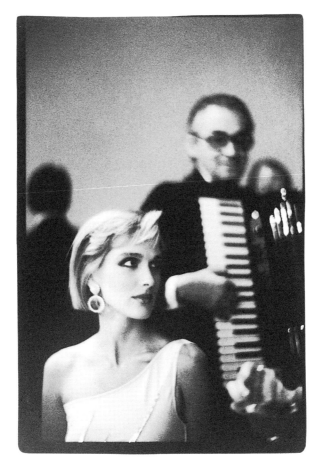

DIANE DEWITT

MARY MACHUKAS

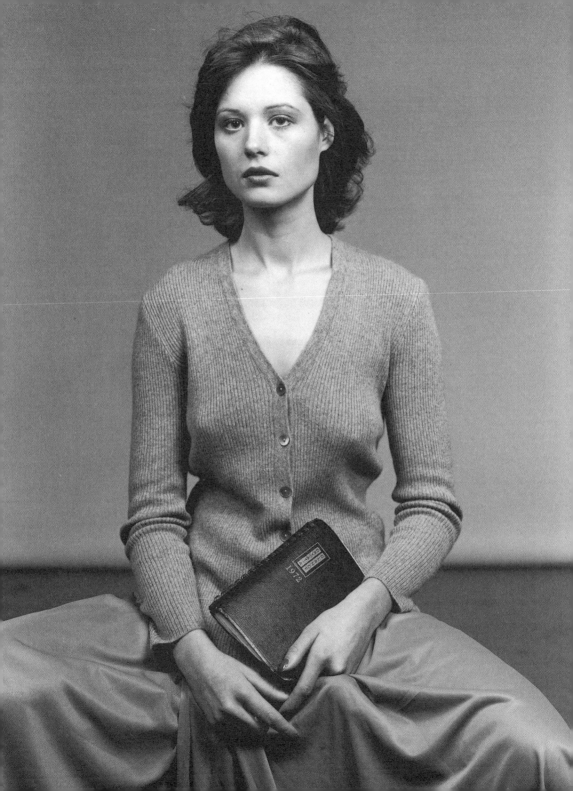

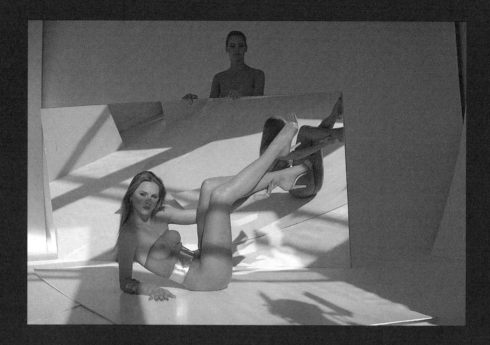

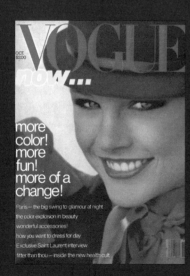

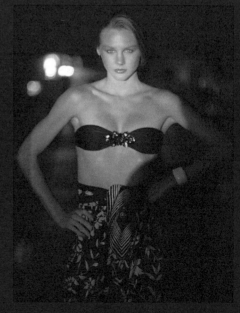

MICHELLE STEVENS

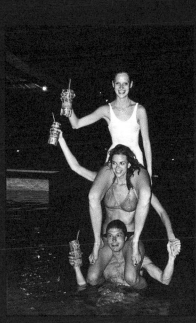

LISA COOPER AND LISA TAYLOR

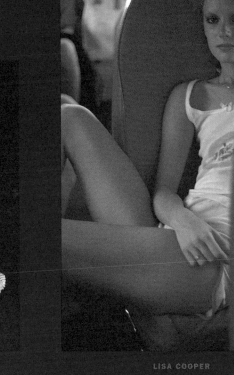

LISA COOPER

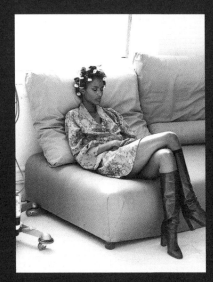

BEVERLY JOHNSON

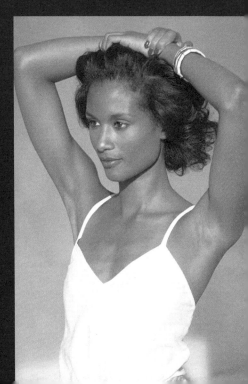

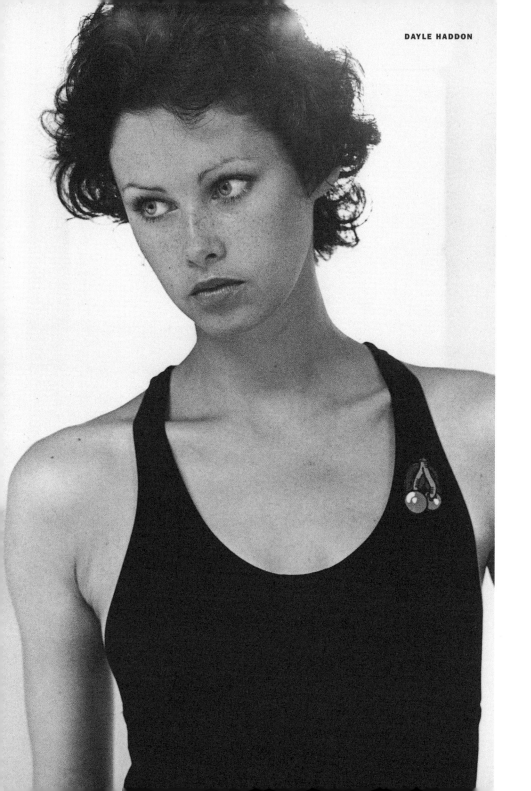

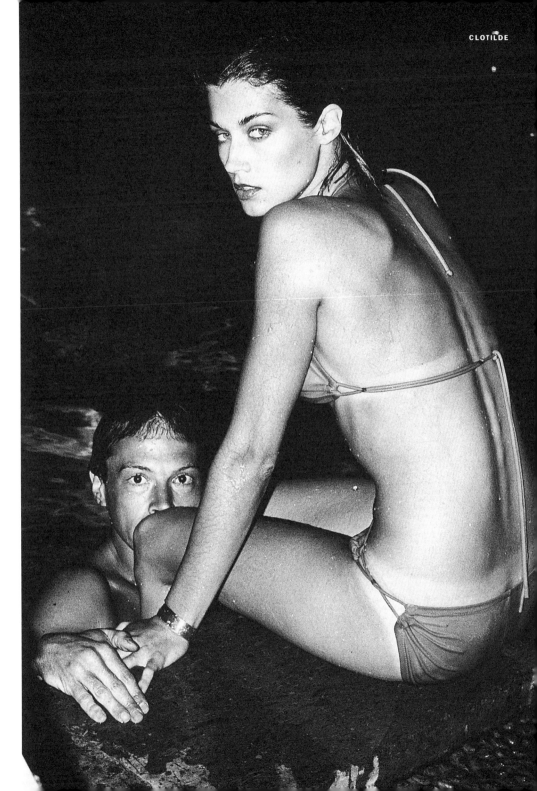

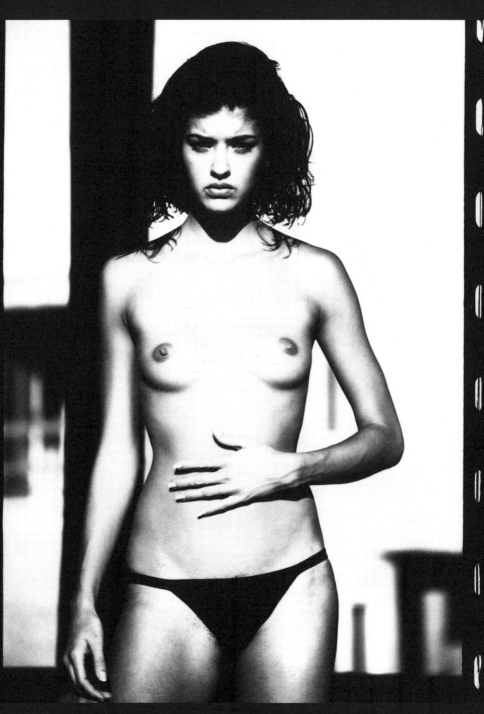

JANICE DICKENSON

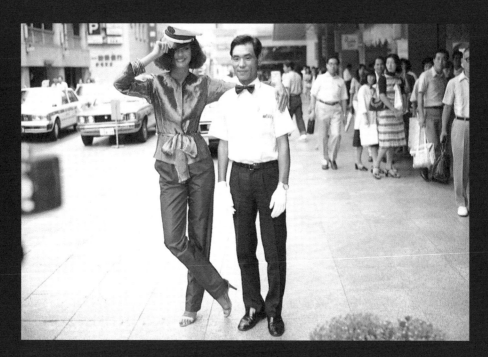

JANICE DICKENSON, LATE SEVENTIES

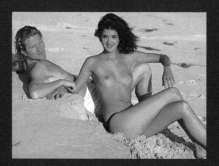

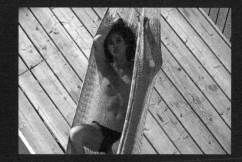

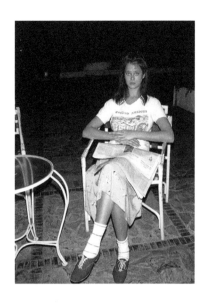

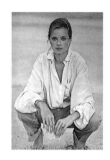

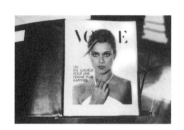

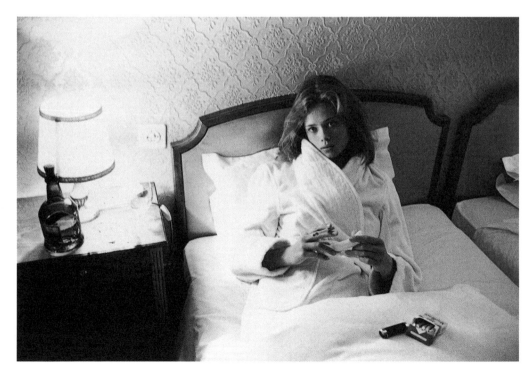

LENA KANSBOD

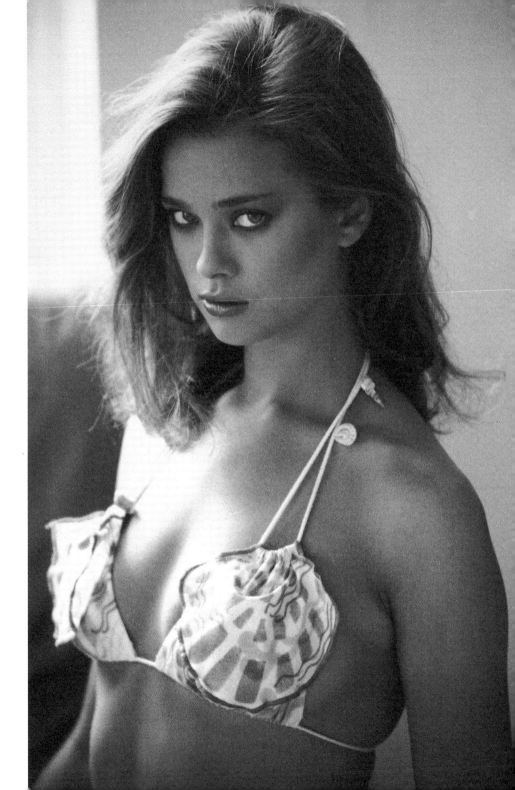

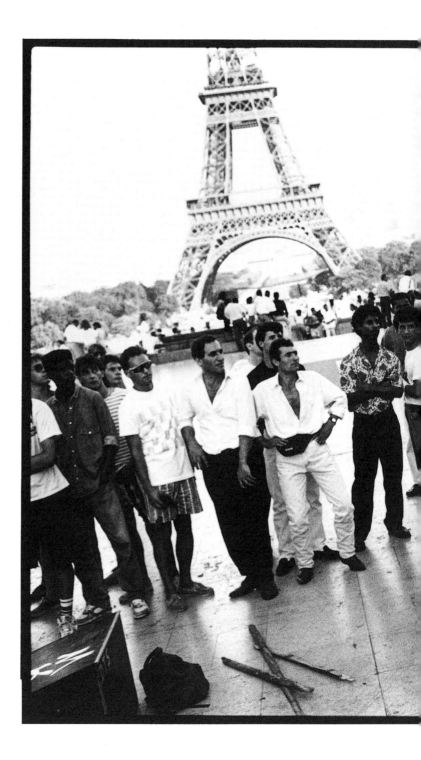

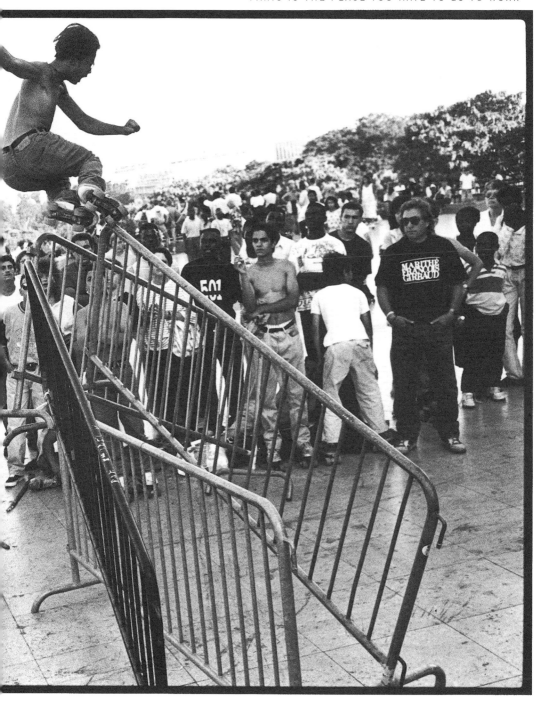

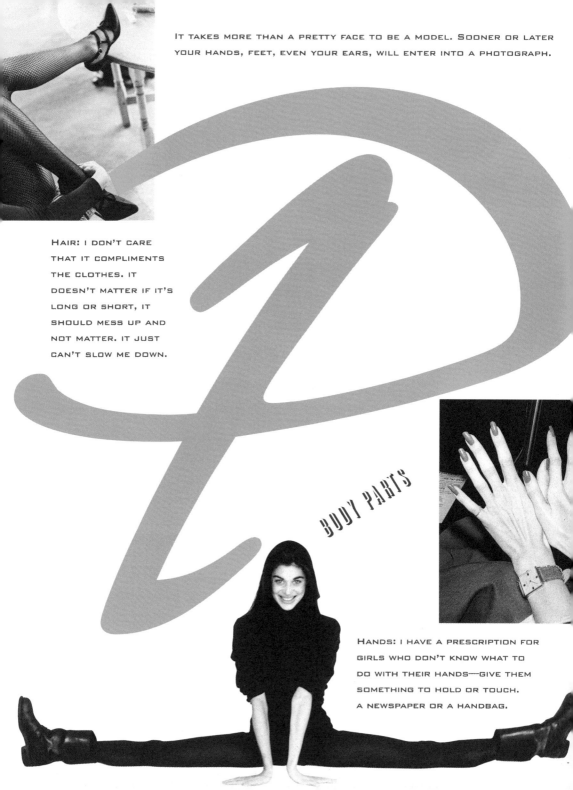

IT TAKES MORE THAN A PRETTY FACE TO BE A MODEL. SOONER OR LATER YOUR HANDS, FEET, EVEN YOUR EARS, WILL ENTER INTO A PHOTOGRAPH.

HAIR: I DON'T CARE THAT IT COMPLIMENTS THE CLOTHES. IT DOESN'T MATTER IF IT'S LONG OR SHORT, IT SHOULD MESS UP AND NOT MATTER. IT JUST CAN'T SLOW ME DOWN.

BODY PARTS

HANDS: I HAVE A PRESCRIPTION FOR GIRLS WHO DON'T KNOW WHAT TO DO WITH THEIR HANDS—GIVE THEM SOMETHING TO HOLD OR TOUCH. A NEWSPAPER OR A HANDBAG.

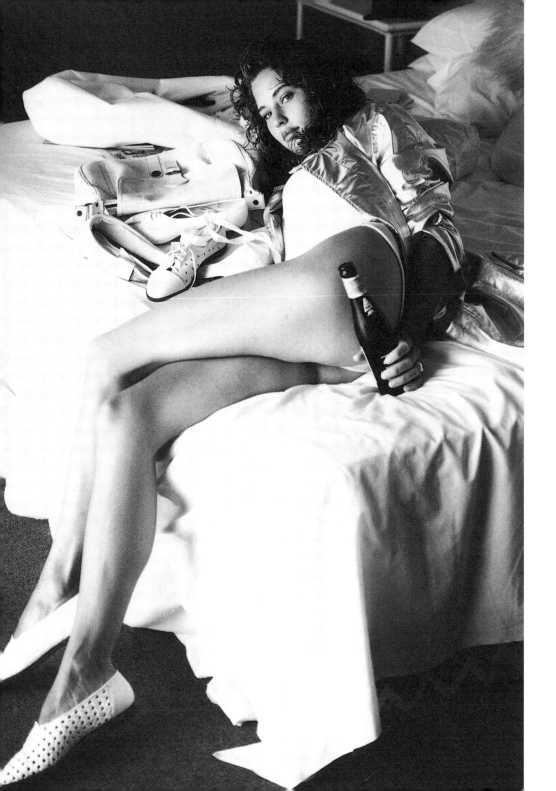

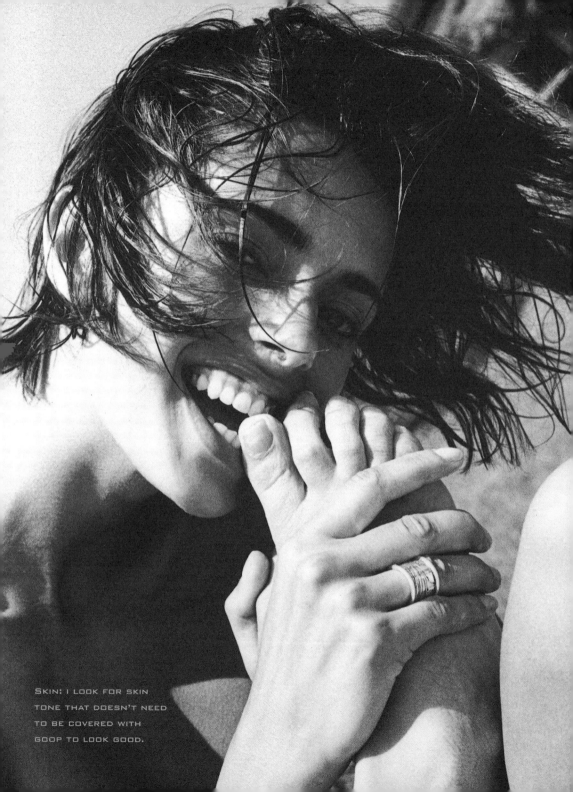

SKIN: I LOOK FOR SKIN
TONE THAT DOESN'T NEED
TO BE COVERED WITH
GOOP TO LOOK GOOD.

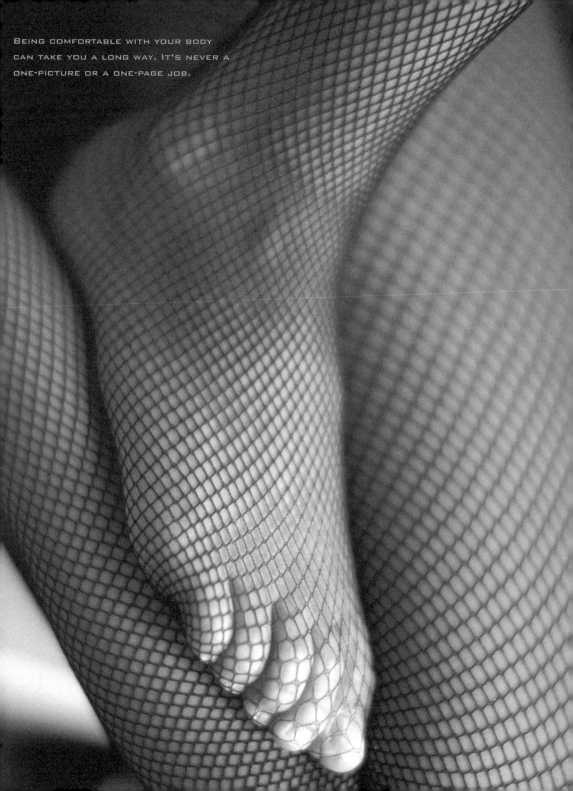

BEING COMFORTABLE WITH YOUR BODY
CAN TAKE YOU A LONG WAY. IT'S NEVER A
ONE-PICTURE OR A ONE-PAGE JOB.

to do after
SCHOOL

Yasmin LeBon is an editor's dream. She looks great in clothes, and if you need her to imitate someone like Jackie O, she always knows exactly what you mean. You just have to find her inner-self and that charm always comes through.

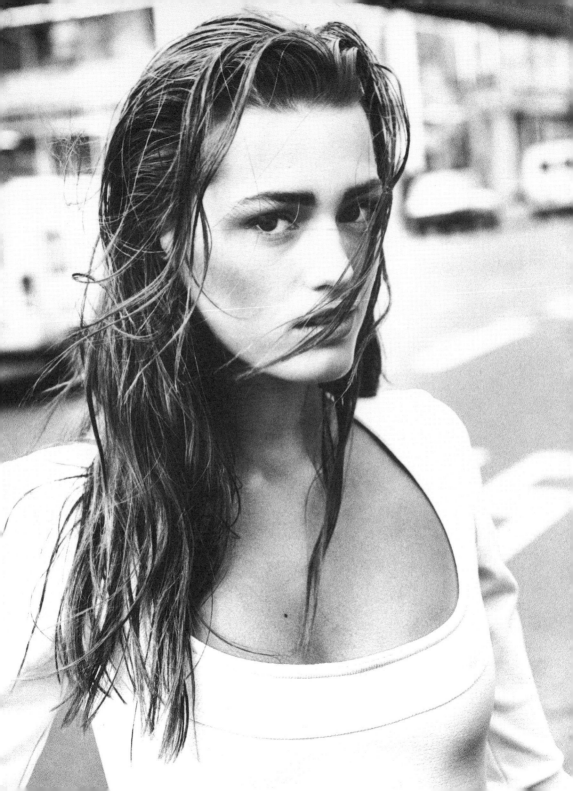

"I never bothered with exercise. I just had a good time. If it meant drinking three bottles of wine every night, then I did."

"With the size of my mortgage at the moment, I'm afraid I'm looking at another fifty years in this business."

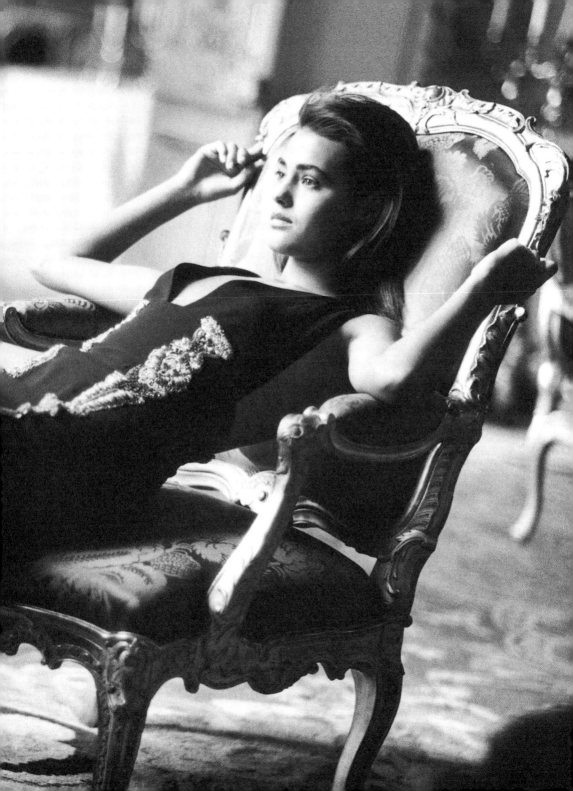

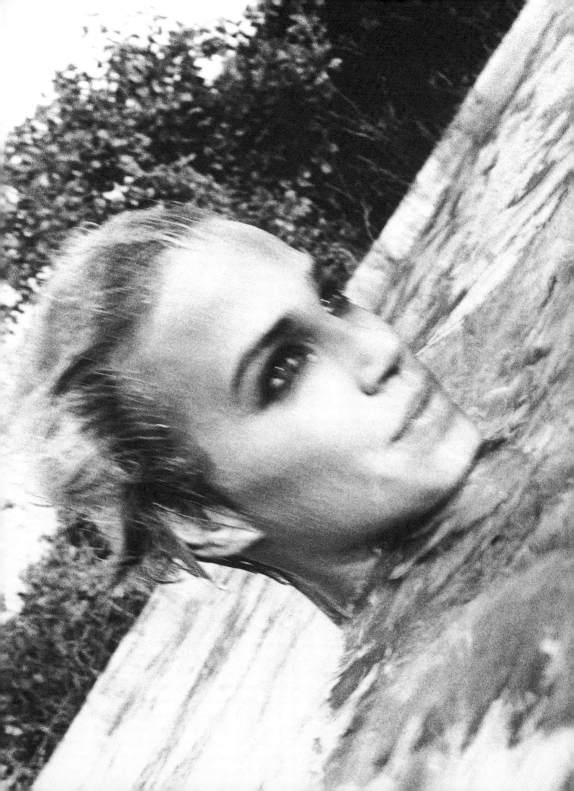

au location

COLOR

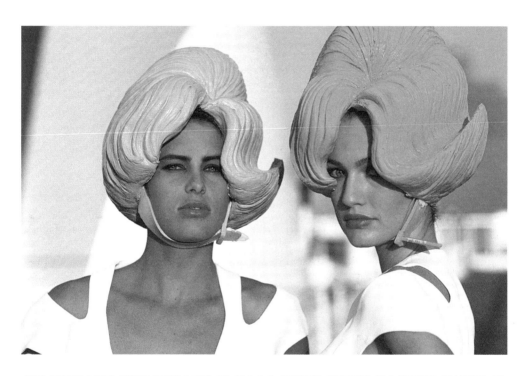

THIS PICTURE WAS TAKEN WHEN I WAS ON THE *S.S. NORWAY,* WORKING FOR FRENCH *GLAMOUR.* IT WAS THE END OF THE DAY, AND I WAS LISTENING TO A CONCERT BY DOROTHY DONEGAN. THE FASHION EDITOR CAME AND TOLD ME TO TAKE A LOOK OUT ON THE DECK. KAREN MULDER AND CARRIE COFFEY WERE WAITING THERE WEARING THIERRY MUGLER DRESSES AND PINK AND BLUE HELMETS THAT LOOKED LIKE WIGS. THE SUNSET CREATED HEAVY SATURATED COLOR AND GAVE THE SHOT AN EXTRATERRESTRIAL FEELING. THE MODELS LOOK LIKE DOLLS.

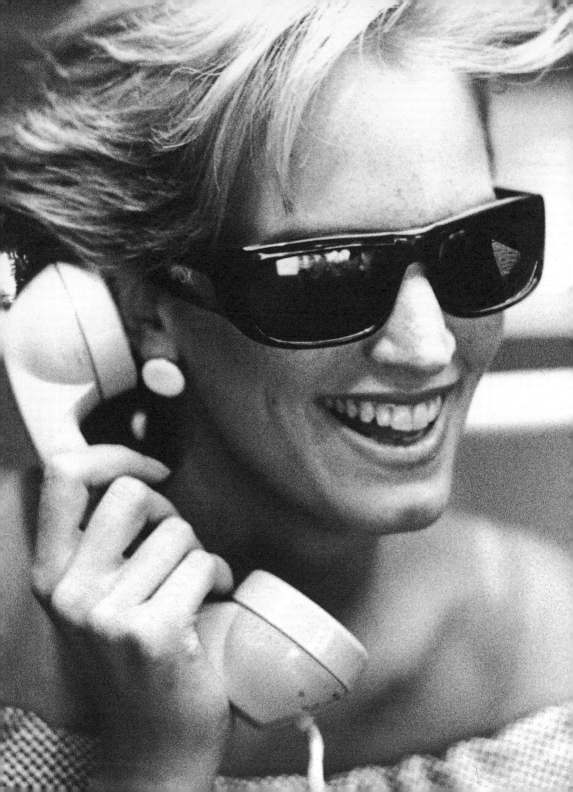

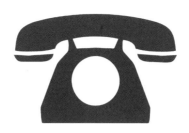

ON THE PHONE

Talking on the telephone is what keeps the models in touch with reality in between shots. It is their link with boyfriends and family back home, but the phone is also the way a model finds out what magazine she's booked for tomorrow and where she's staying in Paris next week. Of course, certain models are more addicted to the phone than others. On one shoot, I had to tell Tatjana not to get on the phone until the sun had set or we'd never finish. And Naomi is never without her cellular phone. I'm happy about the cellular because now *I* can get a phone call once in a while. But I understand why a girl needs the telephone with all that hanging around. And, after all, working the phone is better than working the fridge.

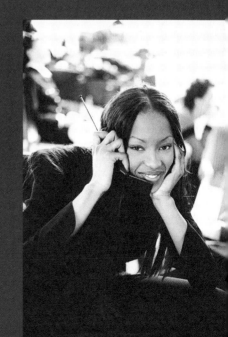

V

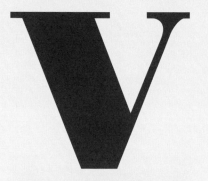

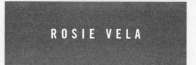

ROSIE VELA

"Now that I'm in front of a camera again, I feel more beautiful and more sensual than I've felt in my entire life. It's just great to see a model who's over twenty-five admired for her beauty. It's also nice to say hello to my old friends."

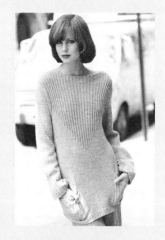

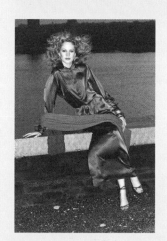

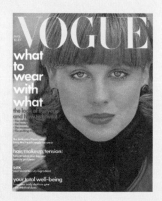

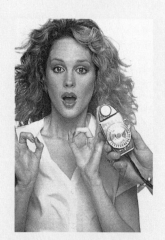

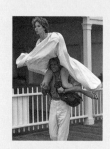

"I came to New York from Galveston, Texas, in October of 1974. I was in my heyday in 1975 and I did my last *Vogue* cover in 1981. It was a wild, heady sensation being on the cover of *Vogue* every other month. It was such an *Alice in Wonderland* kind of world. Back then, the editor considered my top lip too thick and my hair too curly. They would slap on lots of makeup and straighten my hair."

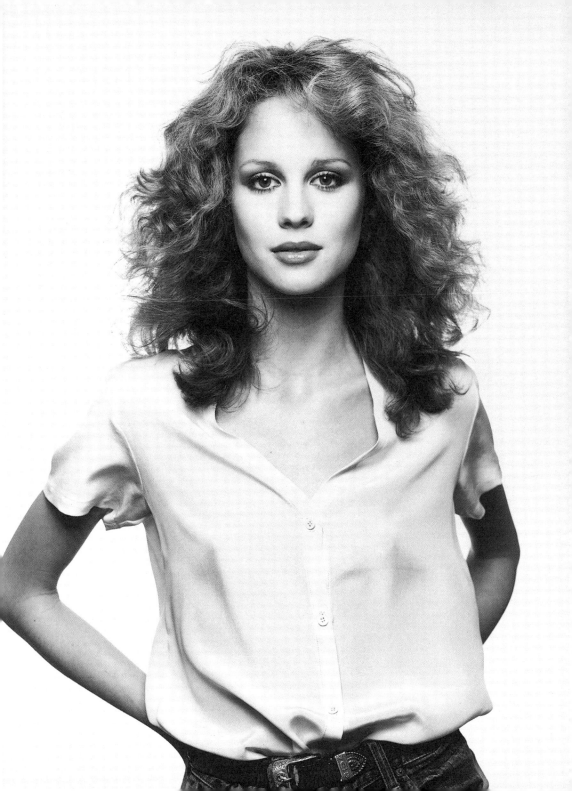

EDITORS

MAGAZINE EDITORS MAKE MY LIFE EASY BY

TAKING CARE OF ALL THE DETAILS ON A

PHOTO SHOOT. THEY SEE THE BIG PICTURE—

THEY COME UP WITH THE STORY IDEA, THE

CLOTHES, THE LOCATION, EVERYTHING. THE

EDITORS WORK WITH ME ON THE SHOOT TO

MAKE SURE THAT THE JOB GETS DONE EXACT-

LY THE WAY THEY ENVISIONED IT. A GREAT

EDITOR SETS AN EXAMPLE FOR THE MODEL.

ULTIMATELY, AS THE PHOTOGRAPHER, IT'S MY

JOB TO MAKE THE EDITORS' DREAMS

COME TRUE.

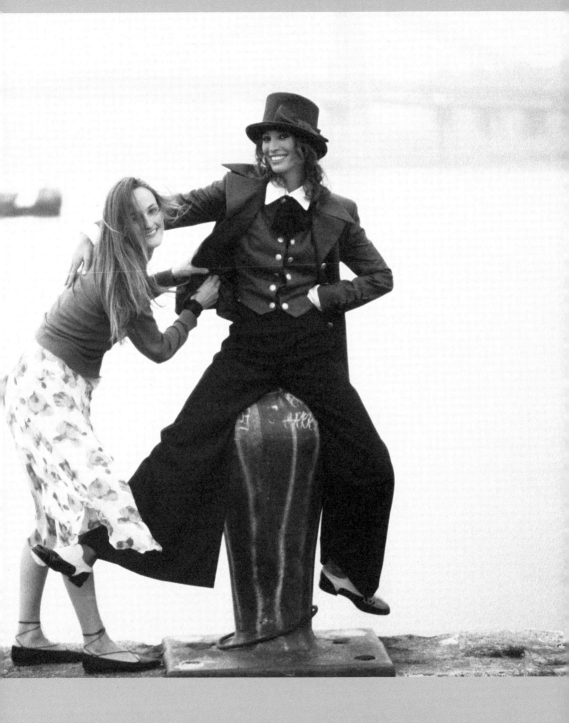

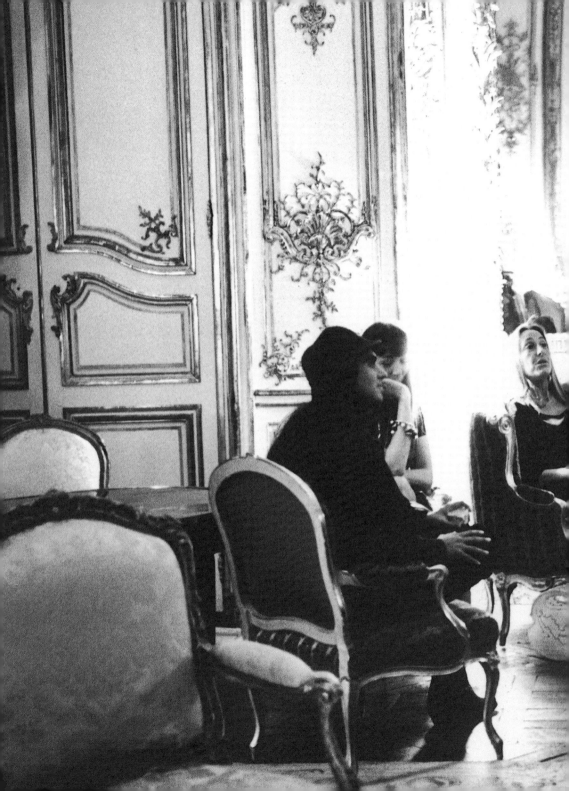

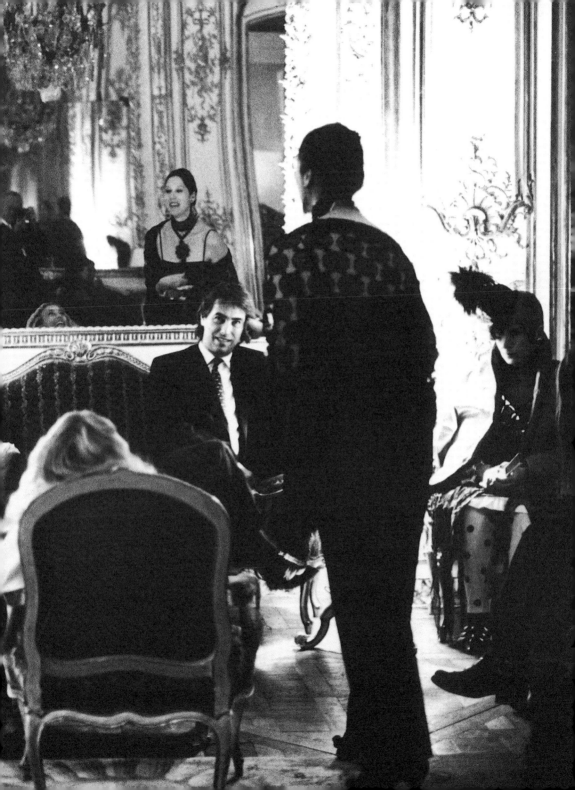

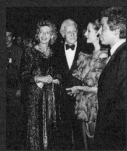

GRACE MIRABELLA, WILLIAM CAHAN

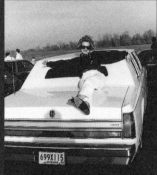

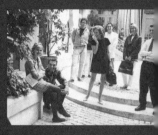

ANGELICA BLECHSCMIDT AND EDGAR OT

SARAJANE HOARE

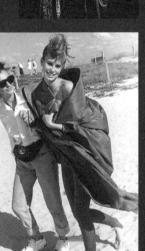

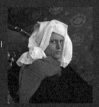

MIMA BARBIERI

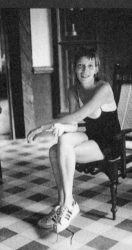

CAMILLA NICKERSON

BRANA WOLF, NIKI TAYLOR

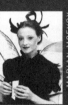

CANDY PRATTS, JENNY CAPITAIN

MARIAN MCEVOY

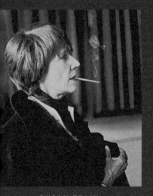

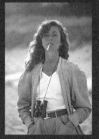

JADE HOBSON CHARNIN

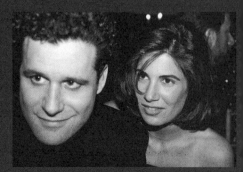

SUSAN TRAIN

ISAAC MIZRAHI, ELIZABETH SALTZMAN

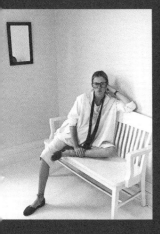

MARY RANDOLPH CARTER

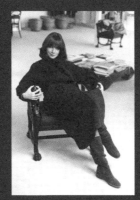

FRANCIS STEIN

THE FRENCH *VOGUEYS*

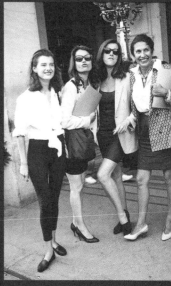

HARRIET CAIN

GRACE, POLLY HAMILTON

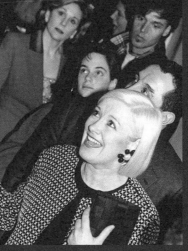

LIZ TILBERIS

BARBARA DENTE, CAROLYN ELLEN

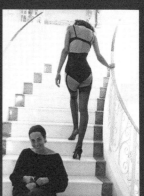

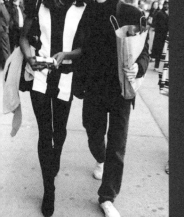

NAOMI CAMPBELL, JOE MCKENNA

POLLY, JENNY AND GRACE

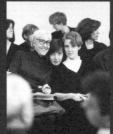

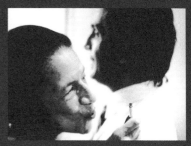

DIANA VREELAND, VALENTINO

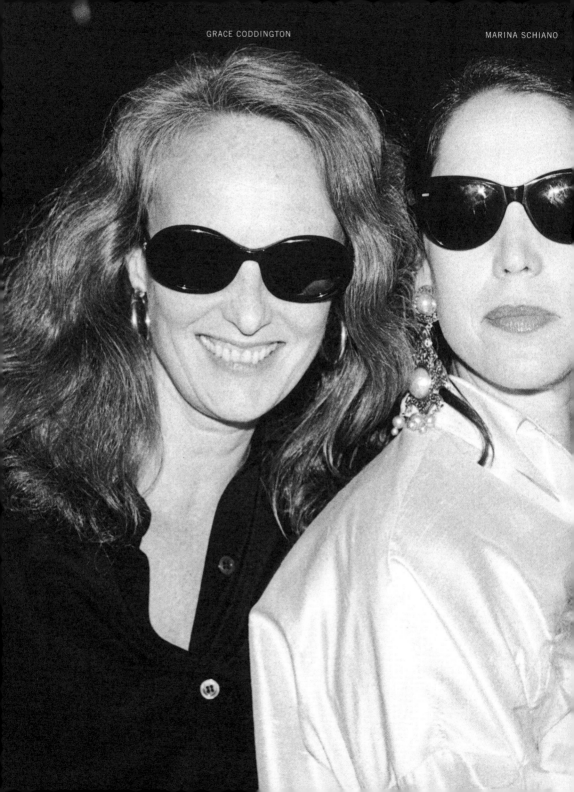

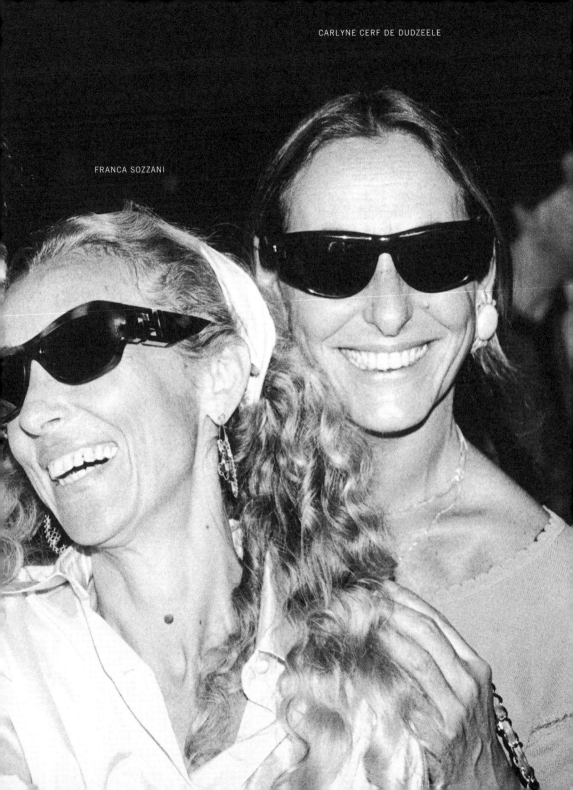

FRANCA SOZZANI

CARLYNE CERF DE DUDZEELE

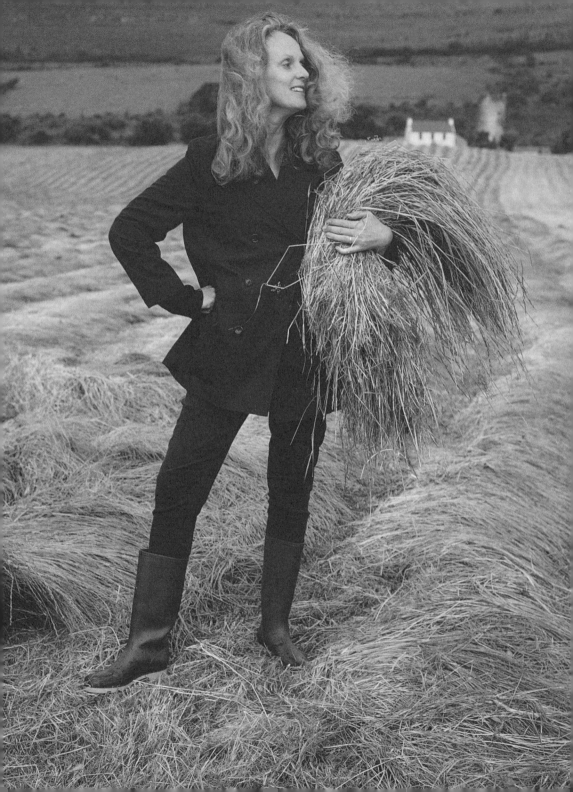

GC

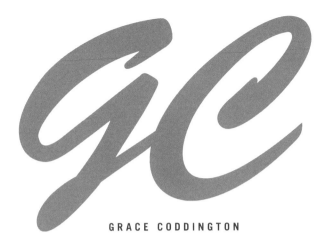

GRACE CODDINGTON

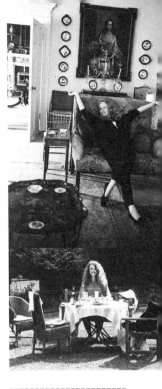

How did you get into this business?
In 1959, I moved to London from North Wales and I met Norman Parkinson. I became a model and worked for nine years. Then I made a neat switch to junior fashion editor at British *Vogue,* where I worked for nineteen years. I've been at American *Vogue* for five.

Where do you get your inspiration?
I get bored just doing endless pictures on a white background. I think there's more to fashion than just a dress and a few necklaces. In fact, I really don't like accessorizing things. My accessory is really the place or the moment, which is why travel interests me enormously.

What kind of look do you go for in a model?
If you start putting girls in a magazine who are going to offend Mrs. Average America then you're never going to sell any issues. So you have to be somewhat safe and do a sort of balancing act. Pretty girls sell, as we know from Claudia and Cindy. Every woman dreams to look like them.

How will you pick a model?
It's very hard. I always look at their books very carefully to find out who they've been working with so I can get some indication of what kind of person they are as much as how pretty they are. You can also check up with Karl or whoever if they've been on the runway, who might say, "Yeah, she looks good but is impossible to fit because she has a short waist" or something.

So who have been your favorites?
Talisa Soto was very special, and I kind of felt like her mother because I worked with her when she was fourteen. I loved Apollonia, who was crazy. Very real. Of the older ones, I think Esmé was very beautiful. And Uma Thurman, Christy, Linda and Naomi, of course. Donna Mitchell was magic.

Any advice to potential models?
I think it's a really wonderful job. You can make a huge amount of money, but don't be fooled that it isn't incredibly grueling and hard work. Have something up your sleeve to move on to when it's over...it can be when you're only twenty-five.

"YOU'RE EITHER HAVING DINNER WITH 3,000 PEOPLE OR GROVELLING ON THE FLOOR WITH PINS IN YOUR MOUTH."

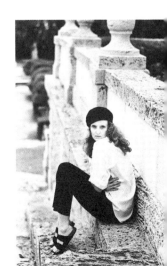

andré

"I THINK OF MYSELF AS NO BETTER THAN A BRITISH AIR STEWARD SERVING 'COFFEE, TEA OR ME.' I PAMPER THE SUBJECT, MAKE HER FEEL COZY, SERVED AND NURTURED. I'M REALLY JUST A PERSON CARRYING A SUITCASE FULL OF CLOTHES. AFTER ALL, WE'RE NOT CREATING THE SISTINE CHAPEL—WE'RE DOING A MONTHLY MAGAZINE. ✴ I THINK FASHION IN THE NINETIES IS IN A STATE OF FLUX. THE SUPERMODEL WILL ALWAYS BE THERE, BUT I THINK THE NEW GIRLS—AMBER, KATE, SHALOM— ARE BRINGING A FRESH ATTITUDE TO THE FASHION WORLD. SOME OF MY FAVORITES ARE CINDY CRAWFORD, LINDA EVANGELISTA, IMAN. PAT CLEVELAND WAS THE JOSEPHINE BAKER OF THE RUNWAY. ✴ MY ADVICE IF YOU WANT TO BE A MODEL: STAY CLOSE TO YOUR ROOTS, ALL OF THIS GLAMOUR CAN LEAVE YOU IN A VOID. NEVER TAKE IT TOO SERIOUSLY. AS BEAUTIFUL AS THEY SAY YOU ARE, THINK OF YOUR FUTURE—LOOK TO WHAT OTHERS HAVE DONE— LIKE CINDY CRAWFORD. PREPARE YOURSELF FOR THE OTHER SIDE OF THE RAINBOW."

leon

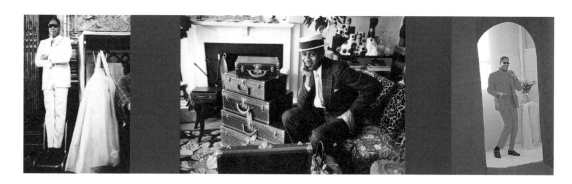

talley

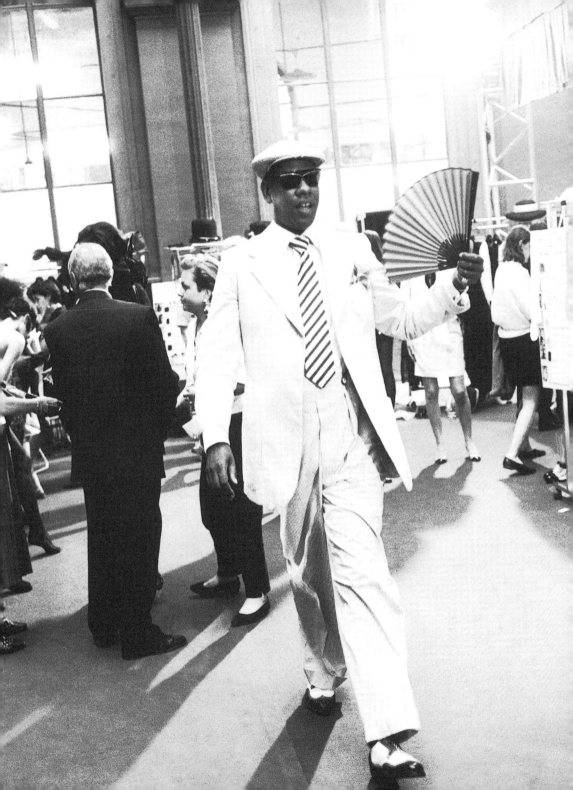

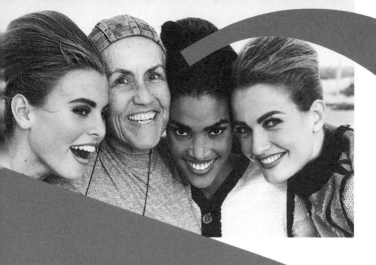

A FASHION EDITOR'S JOB IS TO MAKE A MODEL FEEL LIKE SHE'S THE MOST BEAUTIFUL GIRL IN THE WORLD. I DON'T LET HER IN FRONT OF THE CAMERA UNTIL SHE DOES.

"I'M THE OLDEST LIVING FASHION SITTINGS EDI-TOR IN THE WORLD. I WAS AT *VOGUE* FOR TWENTY-EIGHT YEARS. I'VE SEEN THE WORLD. I WAS PACKED IN COTTON. I'M THE SPOILED BRAT OF ALL TIME."

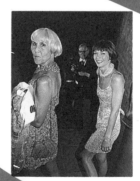

"I WORKED WITH MISS VREELAND AT *BAZAAR* IN THE FIFTIES, THEN LATER AT *VOGUE*, WHERE I STARTED IN 1952. ABOUT MODELS, SHE ALWAYS SAID, 'IF YOUR NECK IS LONG, AND YOUR LEGS ARE LONG THEN WHAT FALLS IN BETWEEN WILL BE ALRIGHT.'"

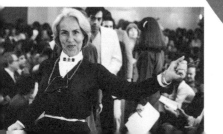

POLLY MELLEN

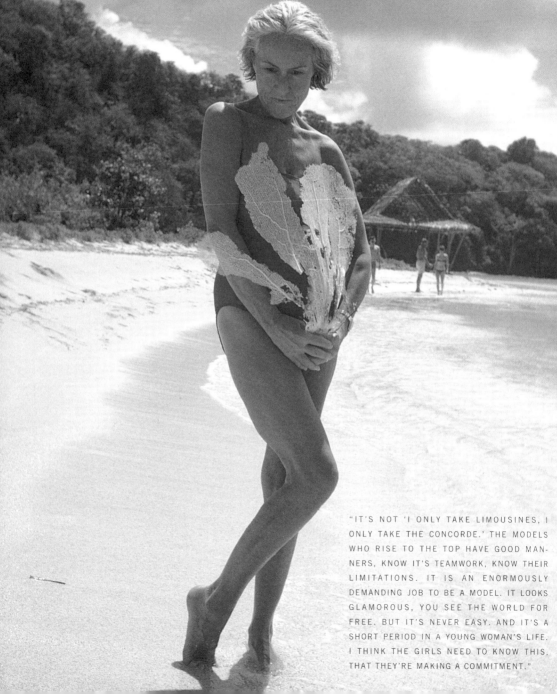

"IT'S NOT 'I ONLY TAKE LIMOUSINES, I ONLY TAKE THE CONCORDE.' THE MODELS WHO RISE TO THE TOP HAVE GOOD MANNERS, KNOW IT'S TEAMWORK, KNOW THEIR LIMITATIONS. IT IS AN ENORMOUSLY DEMANDING JOB TO BE A MODEL. IT LOOKS GLAMOROUS, YOU SEE THE WORLD FOR FREE. BUT IT'S NEVER EASY. AND IT'S A SHORT PERIOD IN A YOUNG WOMAN'S LIFE. I THINK THE GIRLS NEED TO KNOW THIS, THAT THEY'RE MAKING A COMMITMENT."

"**Models don't happen over night. You have to work on them a bit.**"

Grace Coddington

"**Christy is a perfect model. She is chic inside, she has charm. She reminds me of Audrey Hepburn.**"

Carlyne Cerf de Dudzeele

"**A supermodel like Christy Turlington can be a chameleon. She's more like an actress who can play any role.**"

Polly Mellen

"**Linda, Christy and Shalom bridged the gap between looking good in a dress and performing in front of the camera.**"

"I always like the girls who were a little on the edge, like Jeny Howorth. You could put anything on her and she would look wonderful. I love the European girls."

Brana Wolf

"Helena Christensen is totally sexy."

Carlyne Cerf de Dudzeele

"Cover girls are more than beautiful. They have that come-hither face. It comes from the eyes."

Polly Mellen

"NAOMI HAS THE BEST BODY I'VE EVER SEEN IN MY LIFE."

Carlyne Cerf de Dudzeele

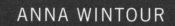
ANNA WINTOUR

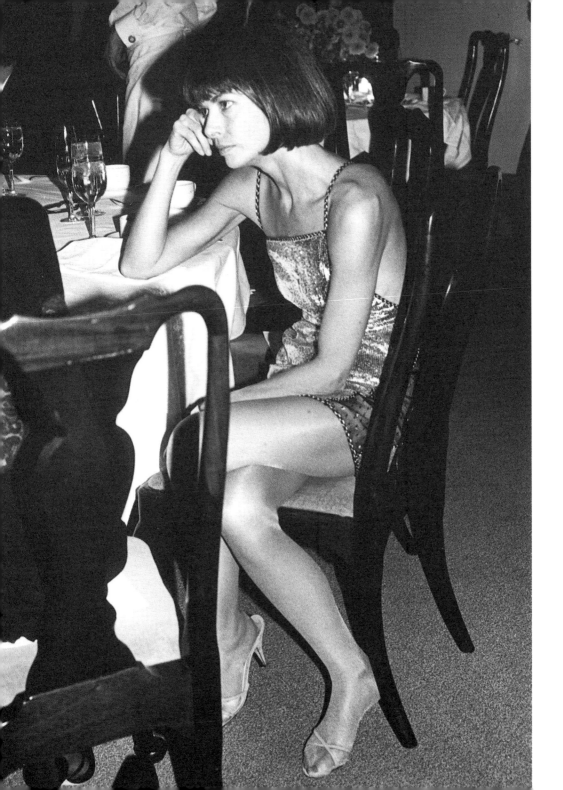

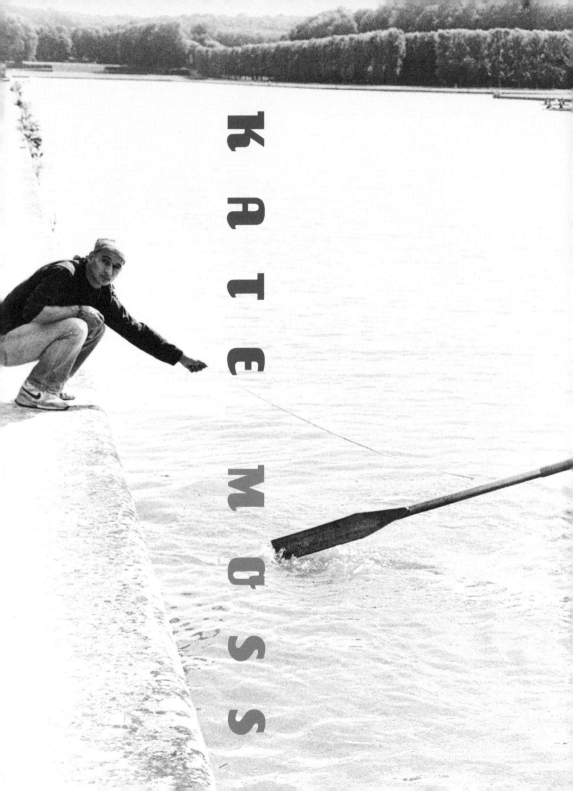

KATE MOSS

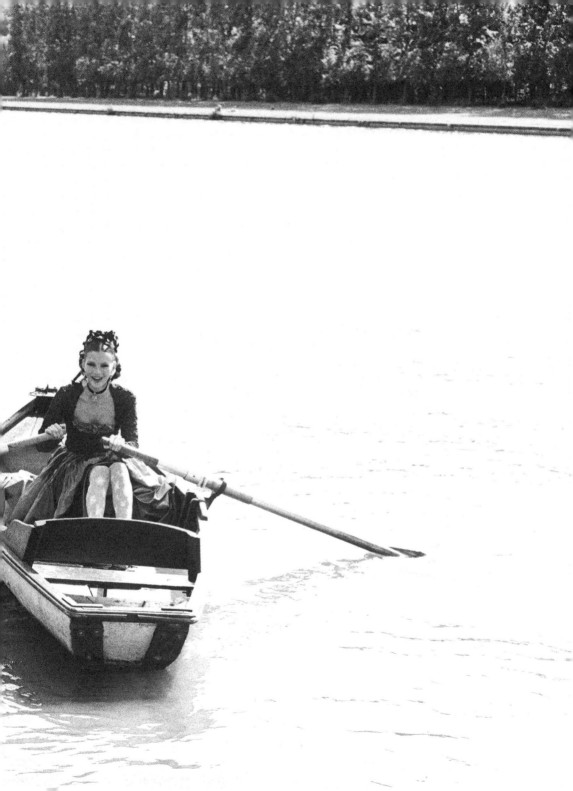

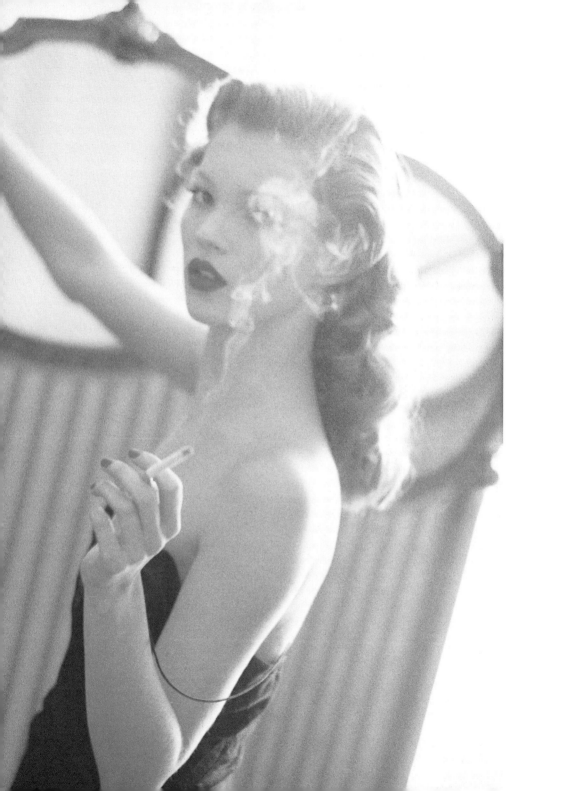

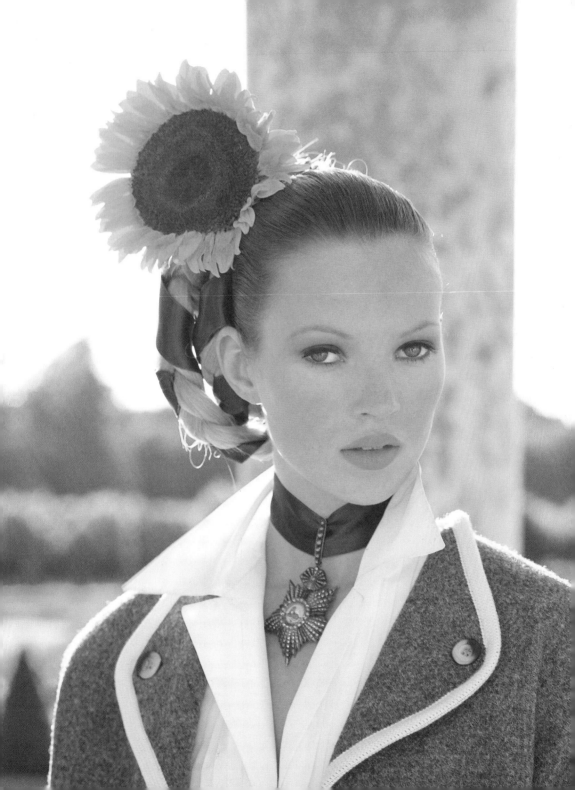

JULIA ROBERTS

BEYOND MODELING

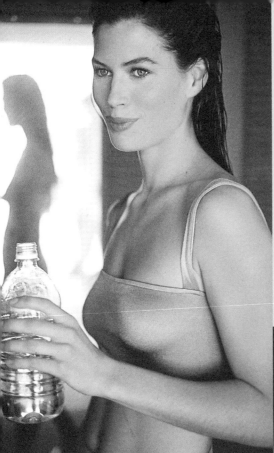

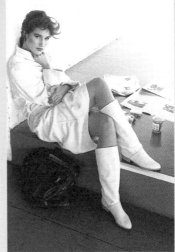

CARRÉ OTIS

ANDIE MCDOWELL

IT'S A FINE LINE WHICH IS CROSSED AND BLURRED ALL THE TIME

SOME MODELS BECOME ACTRESSES, SOME ACTRESSES MODEL,

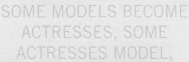

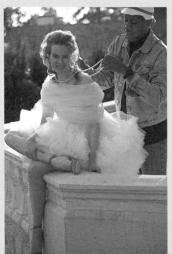

NICOLE KIDMAN

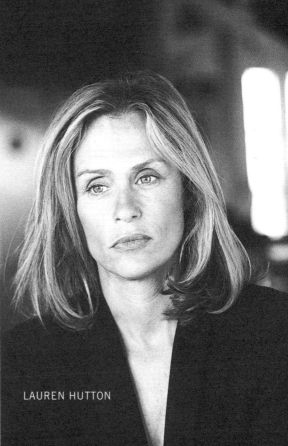

LAUREN HUTTON

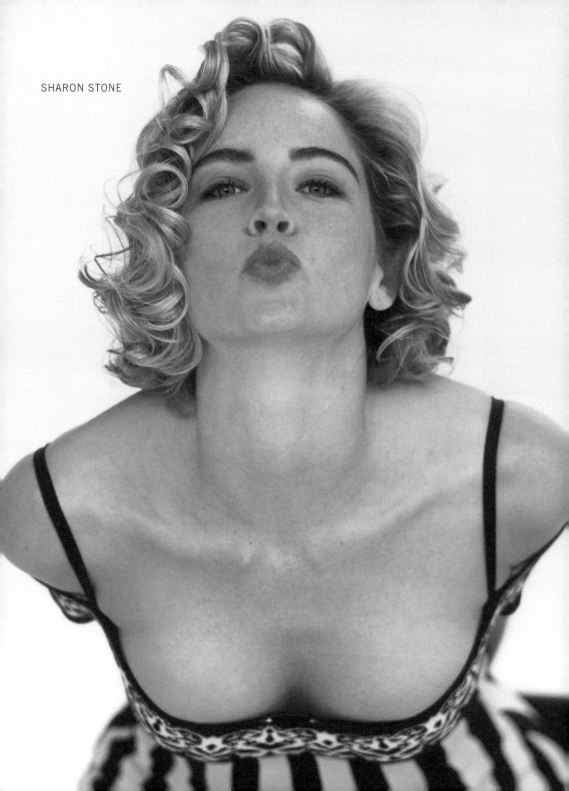
SHARON STONE

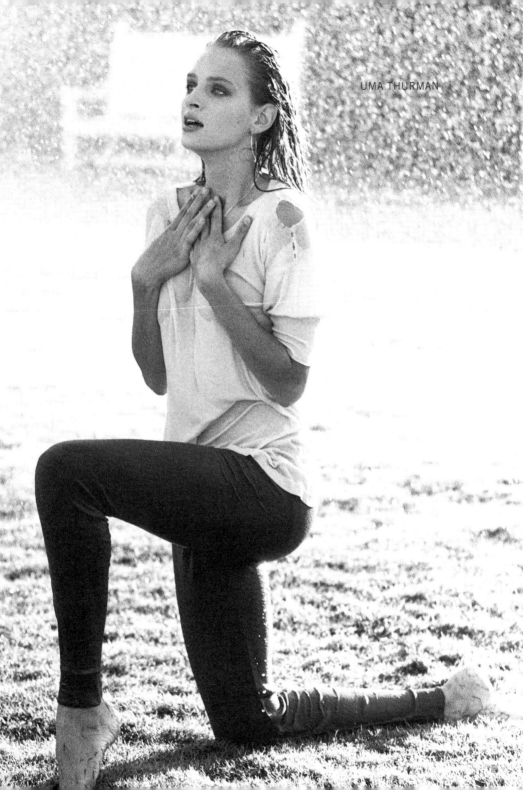

UMA THURMAN

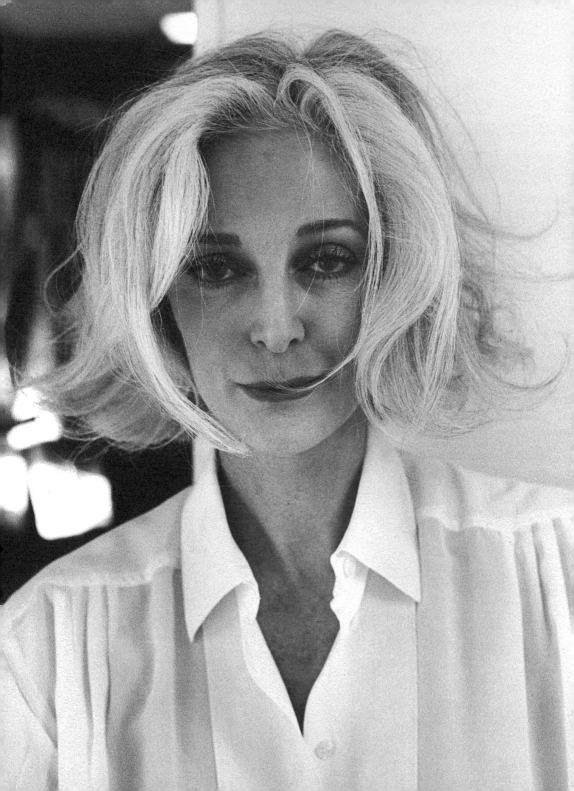

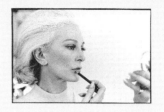

CARMEN

When did you start your second career? I got back into modeling in 1978, when Norman Parkinson asked me to do something for French *Vogue*. He told me I didn't look so bad for an old bag. *How did you get your start the first time around?* I came to modeling accidentally. The only socially acceptable jobs for women were teaching or nursing. If you were esoteric, you became an actress. I had no training. I was very young and poor. *What was your first shoot?* The first day I worked was in 1945. I had seven full pages in *Vogue* wearing clothes by the designer Mainboucher. *How is modeling different today from the way it was when you first started?* I'm part of a different era. There wasn't as much commercial work as there is today. If you did editorial work, you were not supposed to do commercial work. I made very little money, but it was big in proportion to the life my mother and I were living. Peanuts compared to today—back then *Vogue* paid $7.50 an hour. *What photographers did you work with?* All the great ones...Cecil Beaton, Horst, Skrebneski, Penn, Diane Arbus. They loved women in a very special way. *What's the secret of your success?* I've managed to stay in this for forty-five years because I have a well-rounded life and I'm not dependent on it financially. I learned early on how to handle my money. *What do you like about the business?* Modeling has given me autonomy. I've never had to be a slave to an office. It's allowed me to travel. I saw the world before jet airplanes—can you imagine? *Is there a down side?* Today the business is not as much fun—it's dispassionate, uncertain and uncreative. *How do you feel about clothes?* I'm not a slave to fashion. I don't wear bellbottoms. *How do you compare yourself to today's models?* I was never really "in" in the way that Linda Evangelista and Christy Turlington are. I've always been right on the edge. But I have staying power. Before I became known for my gray hair, I was just the brunette with the part in the center. *What was your most memorable photo shoot?* Parkinson and I were on some tropical island somewhere and there were flamingoes standing in this gorgeous turquoise water. I was in a pink bikini. Norman insisted I would look fabulous in amongst the birds. "Just go in there and be a pink flamingo," he said. Well, the water was full of bird crap, and I said the only way I would do it is if he would kiss my ass when I came out. Sure enough, somewhere there is a photo of this six-foot-five man with a camera bending over to plant a kiss on my bare bottom.

✳

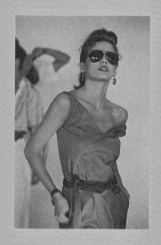

GIA

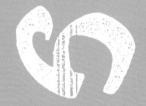

It was the late Seventies and I was doing a catalog for Bloomingdale's and in walked Gia, right off the train from Philadelphia, on a typical go-see. She was tough and streetwise. But I just thought she was a very special face, extremely beautiful, sexy and cool. She was scooped up fast. In fact, that same afternoon the photographer Chris von Wangenheim saw her too. He was so smitten he wanted her all to himself. So goes love for a model.

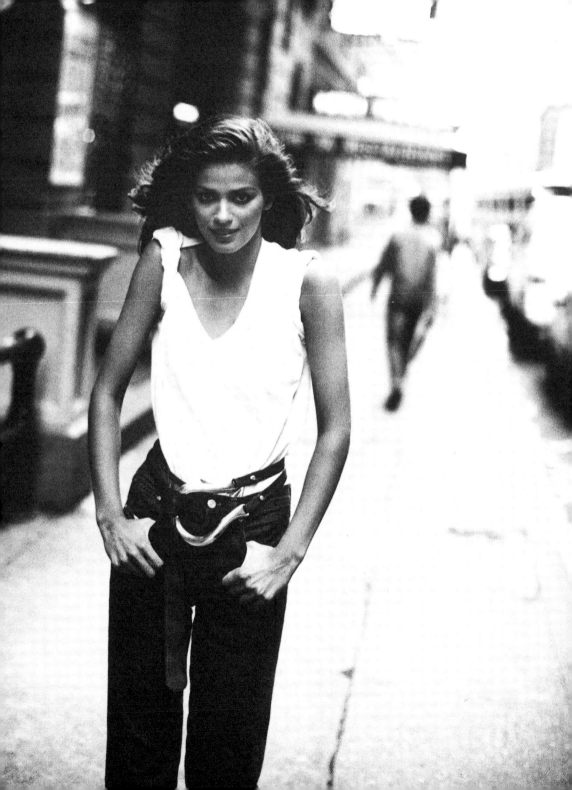

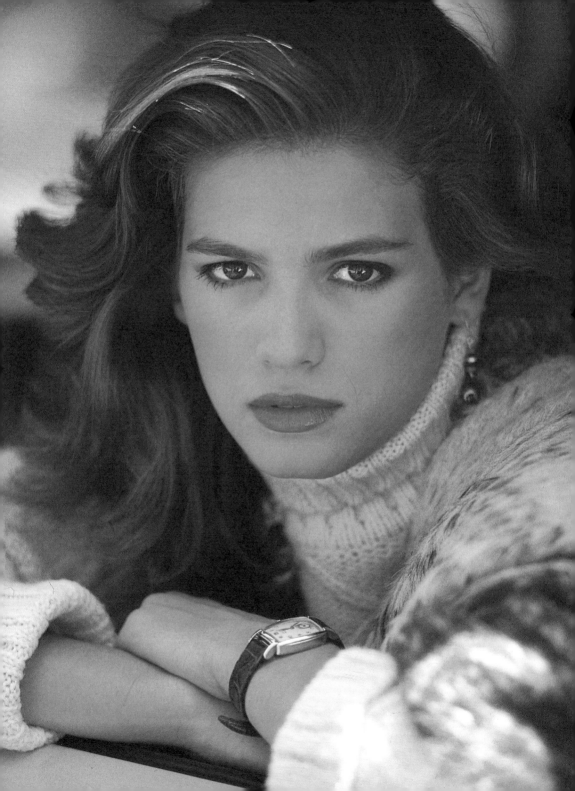

"Gia was fantastic when she hit. She came to town and I thought instantly, 'Oh, wow! Boy? Girl?' I've always been fascinated by Garbo and the way she looked in men's suits. Gia had that same androgynous quality. There was something different about her, a toughness but a vulnerability. I don't know one photographer who saw her and didn't want to photograph her instantly. She was a very special young woman who had a very short modeling career. She made it short because she couldn't handle it. She had a terrific struggle all her life. We lost Gia to drugs." —Polly Mellen

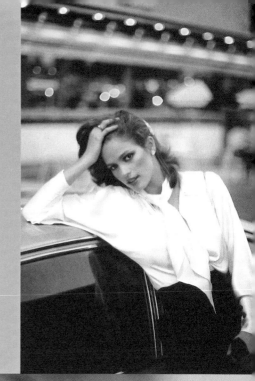

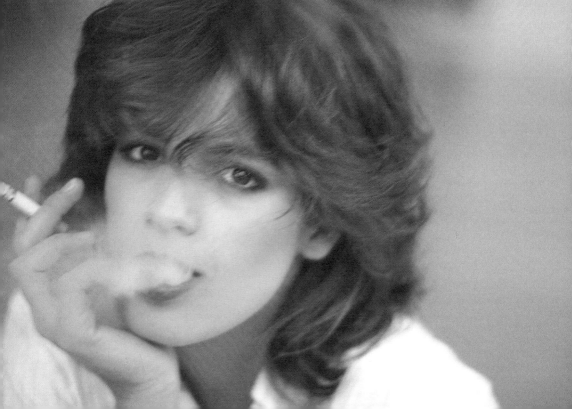

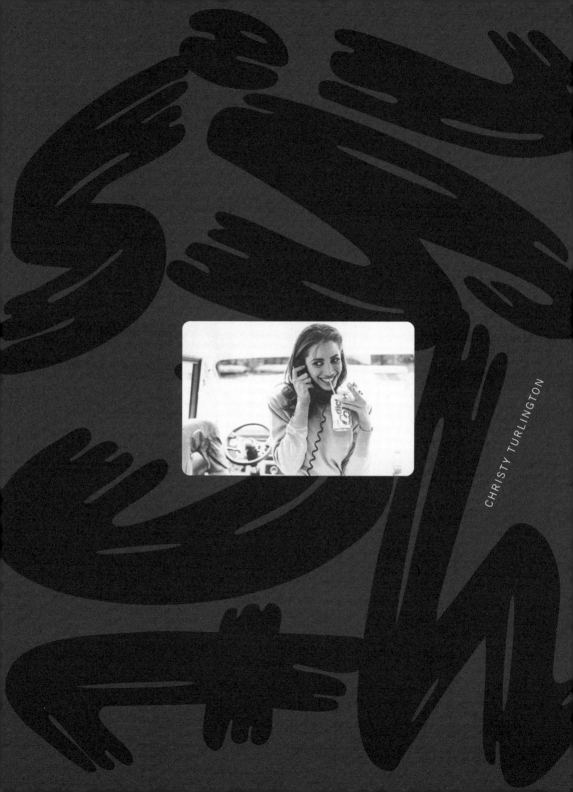

CHRISTY TURLINGTON

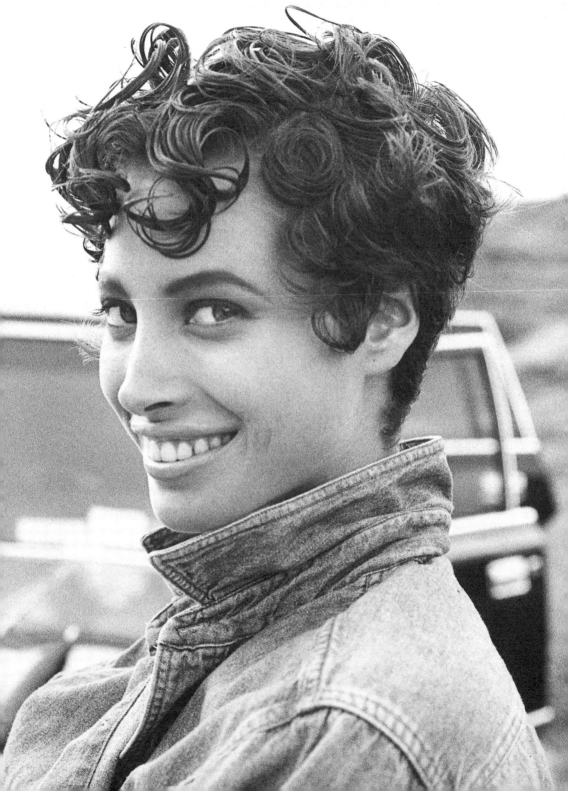

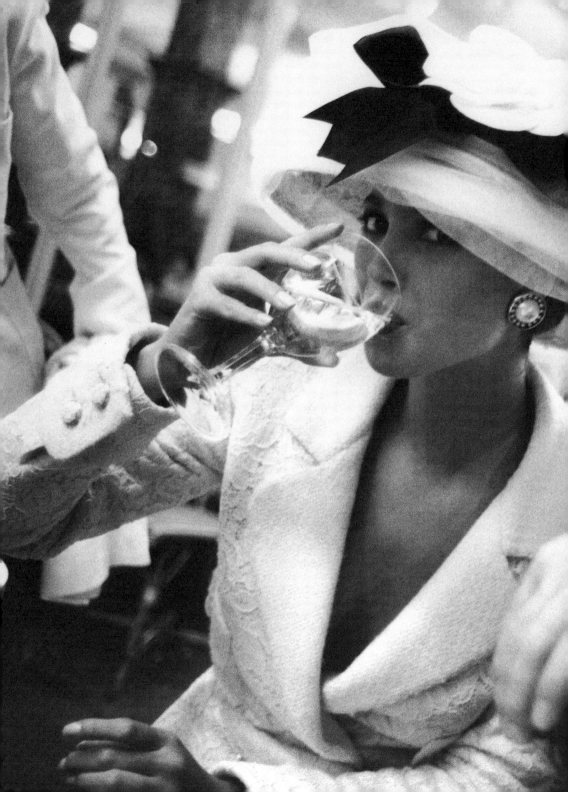

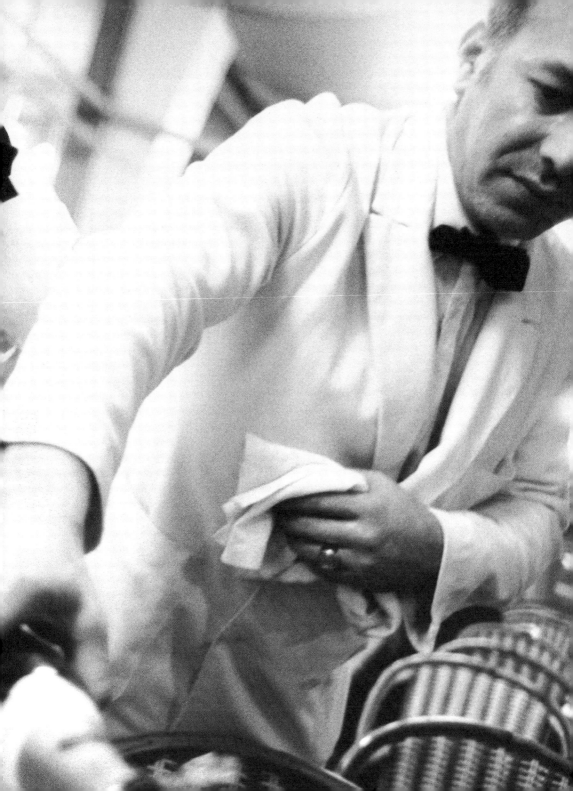

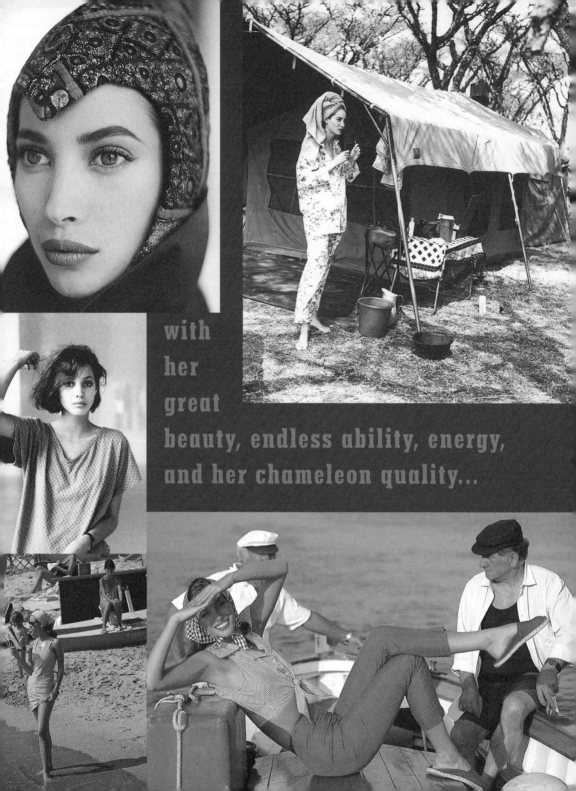

with
her
great
beauty, endless ability, energy,
and her chameleon quality...

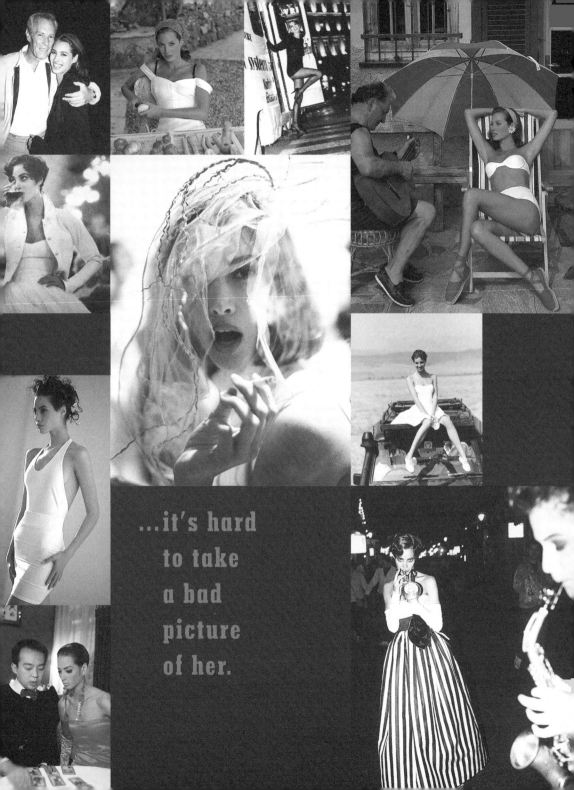

...it's hard
to take
a bad
picture
of her.

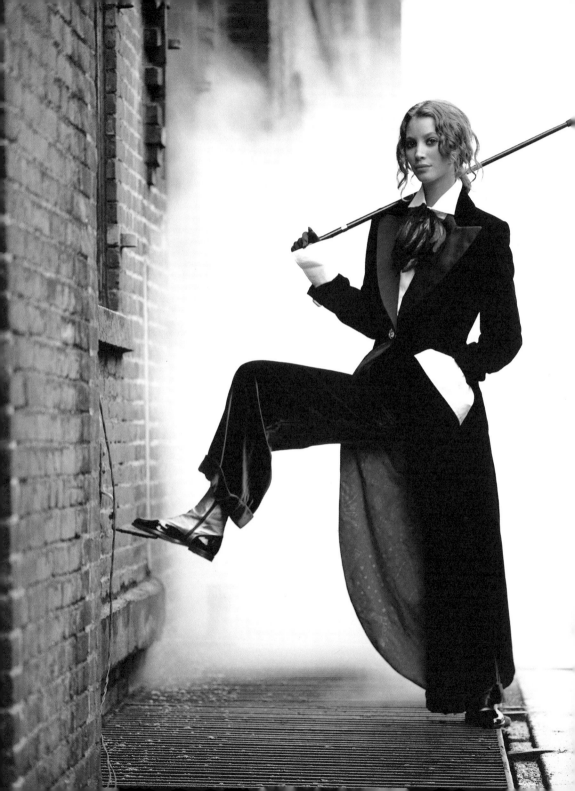

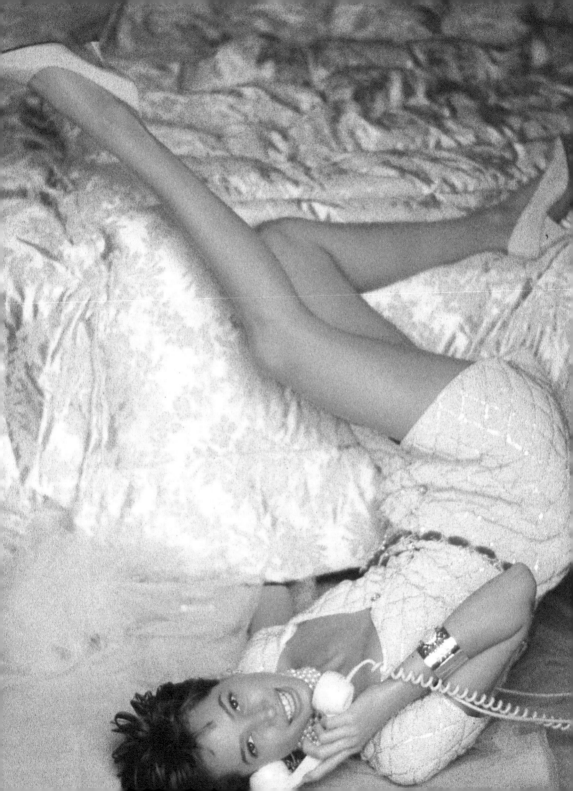

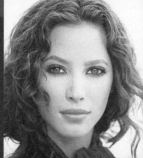

MY PASSION
I LOVE TO RIDE HORSES

FAVORITE MUSIC
EVERYTHING FROM
JAZZ TO R&B,
ROCK AND COUNTRY.

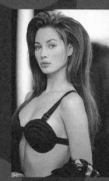

FAVORITE FOOD AT HOME
WHEN MY SISTERS VISIT, WE
EAT BOLOGNA SANDWICHES
WITH MUSTARD AND
MAYO ON WONDER BREAD.

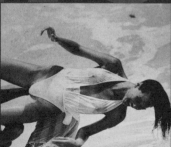

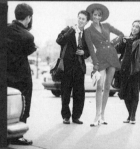

what
nds up
arbage

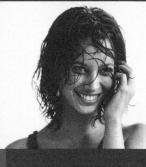

MY BEST LOOK
I ALWAYS FEEL MORE
COMFORTABLE WITH LESS
MAKEUP — IT'S EASIER
TO BE MYSELF.

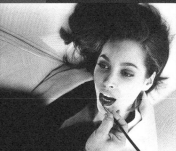

WHAT I KEEP IN MY REFRIGERATOR
AT EIGHTEEN, I WAS FIFTEEN POUNDS HEAVIER.
I WATCH WHAT I EAT, SO THERE'S NOTHING
MUCH IN MY FRIDGE BUT WATER.

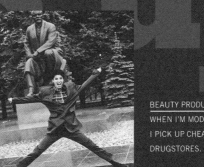

BEAUTY PRODUCTS I CAN'T LIVE WITHOUT
WHEN I'M MODELING IN EUROPE,
I PICK UP CHEAP STUFF FROM PARIS
DRUGSTORES.

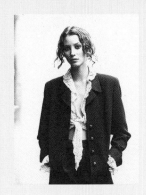

MY FAVORITE MODELS ARE THOSE WHO CAN LOSE CONTROL, WHO CAN ENTERTAIN ME SO I CAN BE A HAPPY OBSERVER, SO I CAN BE A PICTURE TAKER NOT A PICTURE MAKER. WITH CHRISTY IT WAS LOVE AT FIRST SIGHT.

WHAT I DO FOR FUN: I SKI AT LAKE TAHOE AND ASPEN WHENEVER I GET THE CHANCE.

WHAT I DO TO ESCAPE: I SPEND A LOT OF TIME WITH MY FAMILY IN DANVILLE, CALIFORNIA, WHERE I GREW UP. WITH THEM, I FEEL A BALANCE. AFTER ALL THAT GOES ON WITH MY JOB, IT'S NICE TO FEEL NORMAL, TO HELP DAD PAINT THE HOUSE OR WASH THE DOG.

ADVICE TO ANYONE STARTING OUT: YOU HAVE THE POWER TO MAKE YOUR CAREER GO IN ANY DIRECTION. ABOVE ALL, HAVE FUN. DON'T TAKE THE BUSINESS TOO SERIOUSLY. HAVE A GOOD TIME WITH IT.

HOW I GOT MY START: I NEVER THOUGHT ABOUT FASHION AT ALL WHEN I WAS YOUNGER. I NEVER LOOKED AT MAGAZINES. SOMEONE SAW ME RIDING HORSES IN MIAMI, TOOK SOME TEST PHOTOS AND SENT THEM TO AN AFFILIATE OF FORD. I WAS FOURTEEN.

WHAT I KEEP IN MY CLOSET:
I HAVE TONS OF CHANEL SUITS—
I LIKE THE CLASSIC TWEEDS AND
I HAVE A COUTURE SUIT I LOVE
THAT'S RED AND ZIPS UP THE
BACK. I ALSO HAVE CHANEL
LEATHER PANTS, PLATFORM
SHOES AND LOTS OF CHANEL
BAGS. I DON'T WEAR THEM VERY
OFTEN, I JUST LIKE TO HAVE
THEM AROUND. SOMETIMES I'LL
WEAR A PIECE–A GAULTIER OR
ARMANI OR VERSACE JACKET
WITH JEANS–OR I GIVE THEM TO
MY MOM AND SISTERS.

**WHAT I WOULD DO IF
I WEREN'T A MODEL:**
MY FATHER IS A PILOT,
SO I ALWAYS WANTED
TO FLY, TO TRAVEL.
I ALSO ALWAYS WANTED
TO BE A WRITER.

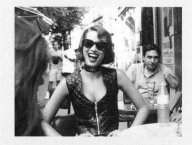

MY ADVICE TO ANYONE WHO WANTS TO BE A MODEL: BE REALISTIC ABOUT THE WAY YOU LOOK. ALTHOUGH HEIGHT ISN'T EVERYTHING, CLOTHES DO FALL BETTER ON A TALL PERSON WITH THAT KIND OF THIN, MODEL PROPORTION. I ONLY WANTED TO WORK FOR VOGUE. THEY HAVE A CLASSY IMAGE. WHO YOU WORK FOR IS DICTATED BY THE WAY YOU LOOK AND YOUR ATTITUDE.

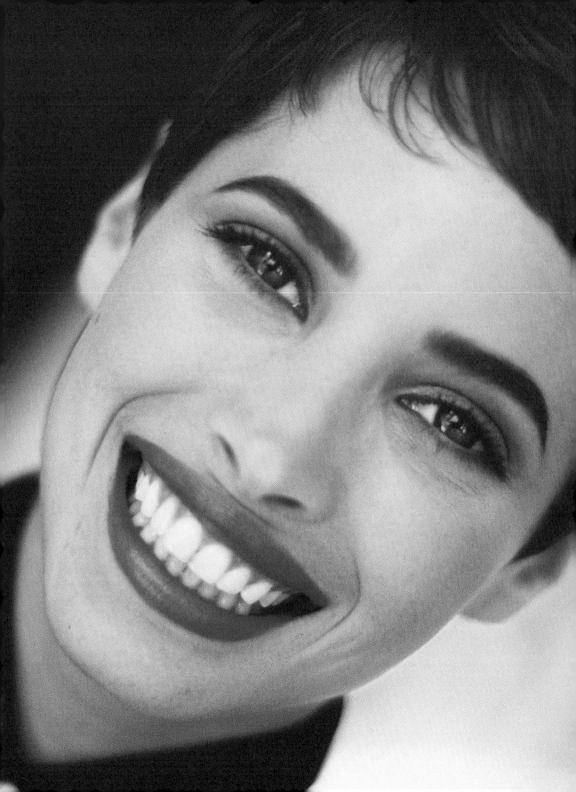

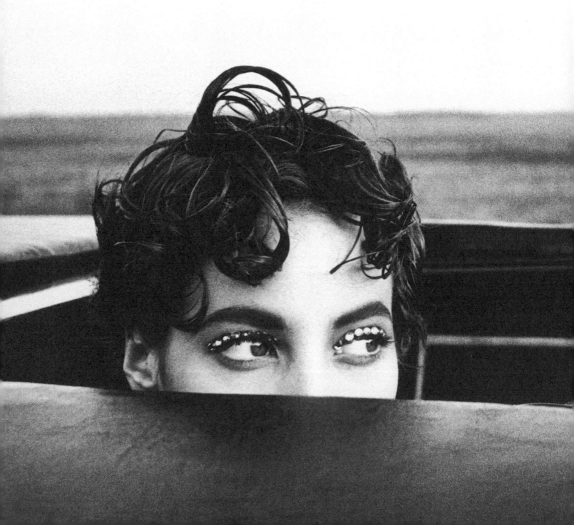

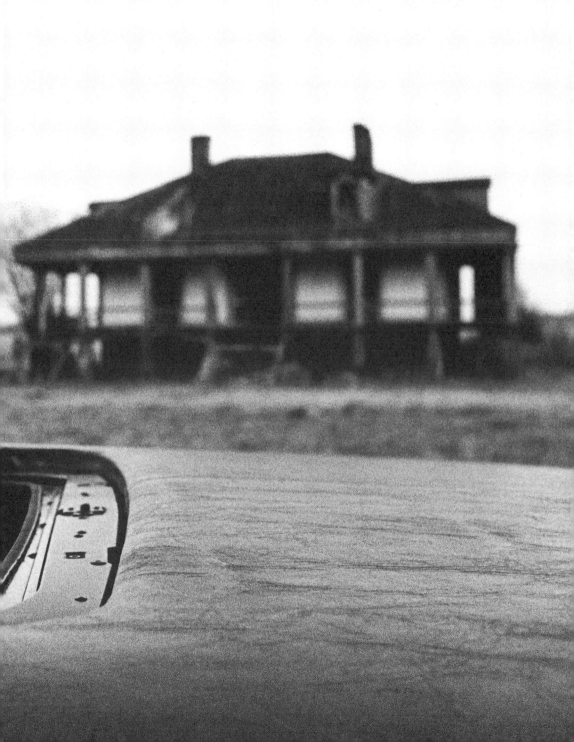

YBE ANOTHER THREE TO FOUR YEARS. I'D LIKE TO GO BACK TO COLLEGE AND TAKE LIBERAL-ARTS COURSES.

"I have the ability to change moods. I don't have limitations. I'm totally open to anything anyone wants to do to me in front of the camera. Most importantly, I never cared about the money."

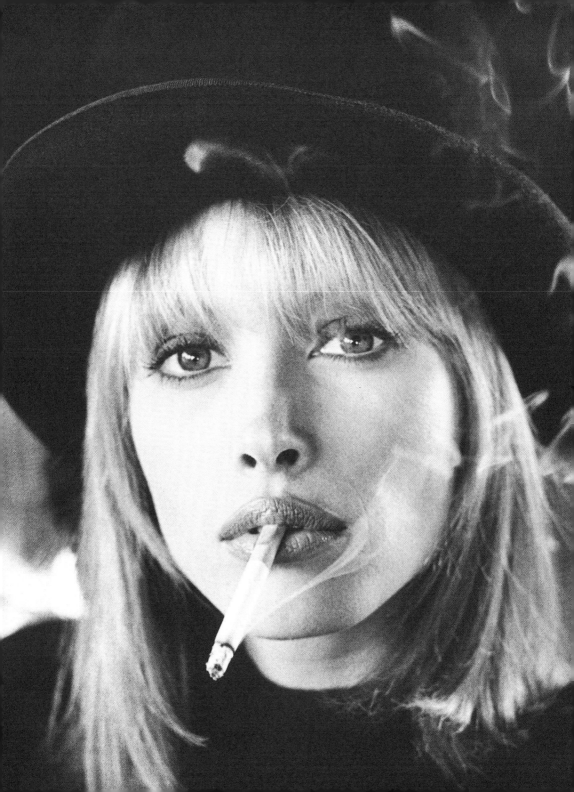

CHRISTY TURLINGTON IS THE MODEL OF OUR TIME

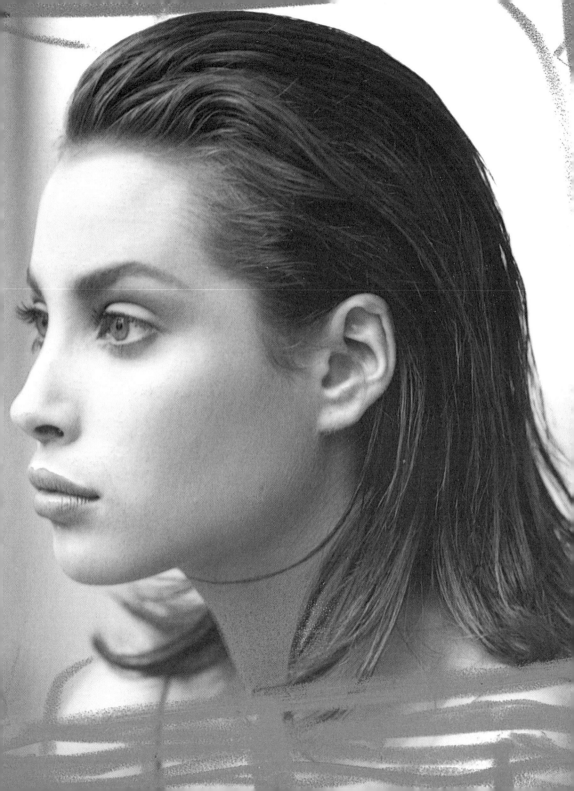

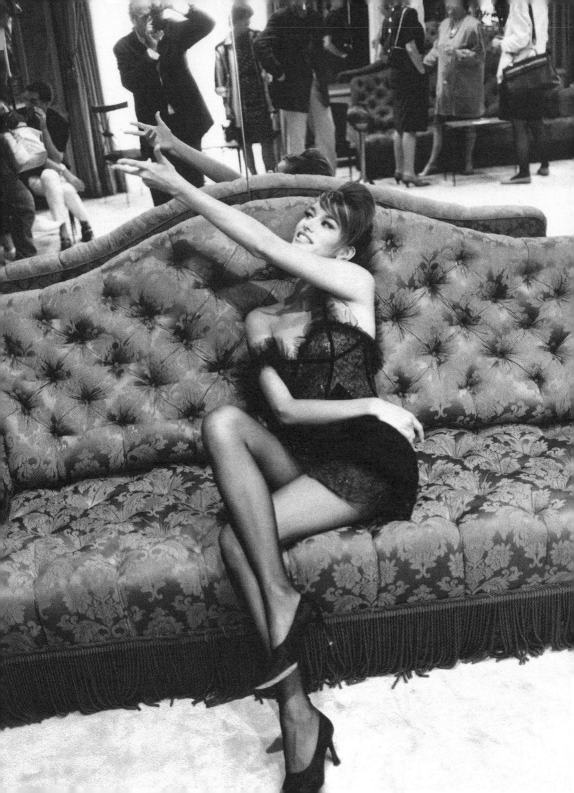

DESIGN
STEVE HIETT
WYNN DAN

edited by

judy prouty

produced and edited by

marianne

managing producer

ron reeves

photographic prints

robert santiago

interviews by

judy prouty

veronica webb

brana wolf

production studio

goodman / orlick design

thanks

Azzedine Alaia, Alexandre, Apollonia, Ariella, Amber, Brigitte Reiss Andersen, Antonio, Ronit Avneri, Nadja Auermann, Emma Balfour, Alda Ballestra, Marc Balet, Way Bandy, Mima Barbieri, Kim Basinger, Barbara Baumel, Nicole Beach, Cecil Beaton, Chris Bierlein, Bonnie Berman, Caron Bernstein, Phyllis Betsill, Karen Bjornson, Billy Blair, Angelica Blechschmidt, Joanne Branfoot, Bobby Boots, Christy Brinkley, Claude Brouet, Harriet Cain, Naomi Campbell, Nell Campbell, Jenny Capitain, Kim Charlton, Carmen, Grant Carradine, John Casablancas, Victoire de Castellane, Anne Christensen, Francine Crescent, Carlyne Cerf de Dudzeele, Cecilia Chancellor, Helena Christensen, Christiaan, Claude, Clotilde, Grace Coddington, Carrie Coffey, Bill Cunningham, Lisa Cooper, Vera Cox, Cindy Crawford, Dalma, Davé, Debbie Deitering, Lucie de La Falaise, Anna Dello Russo, Barbara Dente, Louise Despointes, Diane Dewitt, Janice Dickinson, Peggy Dillard, Kate Dillon, Gabe Doppelt, Meghan Douglas, Gilles Dufour, Anh Duong, Aly Dunne, Gail Elliott, Esmé, Linda Evangelista, Elisabetta Ferracci, Eileen Ford, Juli Foster, Yasmeen Ghauri, Gia, Giancarlo, Konstantin Gonchavov, Francis Grill, Jill Goodacre, Wallis Franken Montana, Mary Greenwell, Madame Grés, Dayle Haddon, Jerry Hall, Polly Hamilton, Patti Hansen, Bethann Hardison, Charles Harris, Patrica Hartmann, Matt Haviland, Sarajane Hoare, Susan Hess, Jane Hitchcock, Jade Hobson Charnin, Maury Hobson, Grethe Holby, Susan Holmes, Tim Holt, Karen Howard, Jeny Howorth, Rachel Hunter, Lauren Hutton, Iman, Elaine Irwin, Marc Jacobs, Jamie, Janine, Jason, Beverly Johnson, Grace Jones, Juliette, Peter Kagan, Lena Kansbod, Jocelyn Kargére, Katoucha, Rei Kawakubo, Amy Kizer, Calvin Klein, Nicole Kidman, Sonia Kashuk, Irina Kuksenaite, Christian Lacroix, Laetitia Firmin-Didot, Karl Lagerfeld, Laurie, Lea, Yasmin Lebon, Abby Lewis Seymour, Gunilla Lindblad, Sandy Linter, Lisa Love, Bonnie Lyshor, Mary Machukas, Robyn MacKintosh, Didier Malige, Gerald Marie, Heidi Morawetz, Marpessa, Andie McDowell, Marian McEvoy, Joe McKenna, Kristen McMenamy, Steven Meisel, Martine de Menthon, Polly Mellen, Misty, Grace Mirabella, Isaac Mizrahi, Susan Moncur, Claude Montana, Kate Moss, Karen Mulder, Nadège, Vincent Nasso, Camilla Nickerson, Chris Nofziger, Serge Normant, Michelle Ocampo, Ric Ocasek, Oribe, Carré Otis, Edgar Otte, Tatjana Patitz, Paulina, Paloma Picasso, Bonnie Pfeifer, Anna Piaggi, Monique Pillard, Pirelli, Emily Potter, Francline Pratt, Candy Pratts, Prudence, Rafael, Mary Randolph Carter, Rex, Julia Roberts, Stephanie Roberts, Romeo, Isabella Rossellini, Renée Russo, Lisa Rutledge, Elizabeth Saltzman, Marina Schiano, Barbara Schlager, Lydia Schneider, Joan Severance, Stephanie Seymour, Marie Seznac, Shalom, Claudia Schiffer, Brooke Shields, Charlene Short, Simone, Emma Sjoberg, Shelly Smith, Franca Sozzani, Stephen Sprouse, Ronnie Stam, Giorgio St. Angelo, Isabella Stanhope, Francis Stein, Michelle Stevens, Heather Stewart-Whyte, Sharon Stone, Theresa Stewart, Annette Sty, Anna Sui, Suga, Suzanna, André Leon Talley, Lisa Taylor, Niki Taylor, Thibaud, Uma Thurman, Liz Tilberis, Cheryl Tiegs, Isabelle Townsend, Troy, Christy Turlington, Mr. Turlington, Tyra, Ungaro, Ellen Von Unwerth, Valentino, Valentin, Rosie Vela, Diana Vreeland, Wendy Whalen, Wendy Whitelaw, Leslie Winer, Anna Wintour, Yannick, Kara Young, Yves Saint Laurent and special thanks to Condé Nast for all the great opportunities.

MORE ROLL!

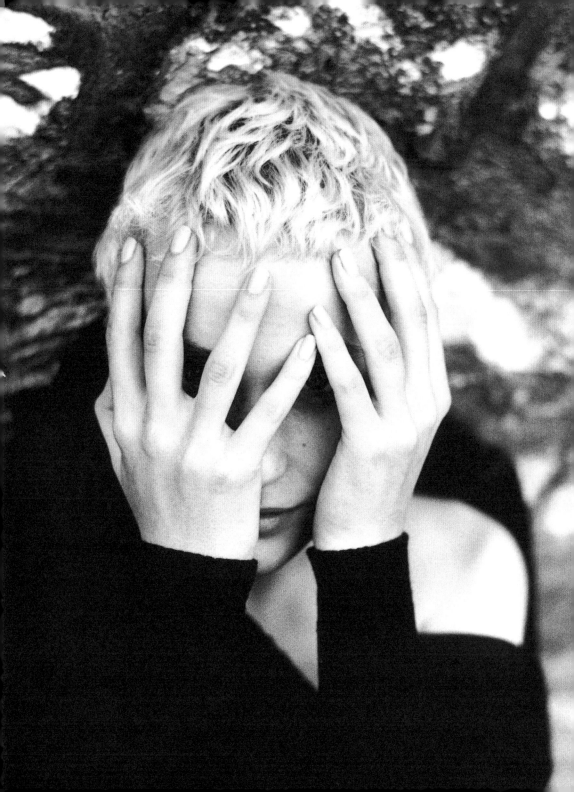

Models into ....

MODELING CAN BE A WONDERFUL AND LUCKY MEANTIME, AND TEN YEARS LATER YOU MIGHT HAVE TO BE DOING OTHER THINGS. START USING YOUR AIRPLANE TIME TO BE INSPIRED ABOUT WHAT TO DO NEXT. YOU COULD BECOME SOMETHING FASHION RELATED, EDITOR, DESIGNER, PHOTOGRAPHER, OR MAYBE AN ACTRESS, RESTAURA-TEUR, GO BACK TO SCHOOL, GET YOUR PH.D. IN RUSSIAN (LIKE BONNIE BERMAN), MARRY A ROCK STAR, HAVE A FAMILY, ETC. LIFE IS GREAT, ENJOY YOUR MODELING AND SAVE SOME MONEY. THINK ABOUT TOMORROW – JUST IN CASE YOU'RE NOT A CARMEN OR LAUREN HUTTON. IF YOU DO FIND A GOOD FUTURE PEOPLE WILL PROBABLY ALWAYS ASK YOU TO BE PHOTOGRAPHED BUT YOU WON'T HAVE TO DEPEND ON IT.

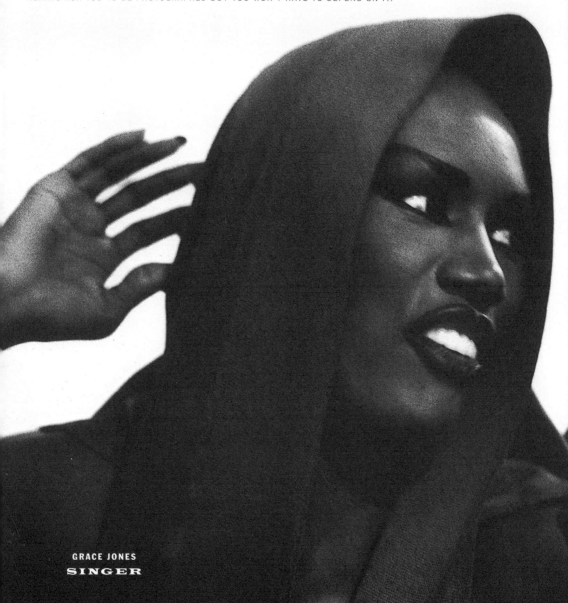

GRACE JONES
SINGER

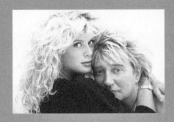

RACHEL HUNTER + ROD STEWART
ROCK 'N ROLL

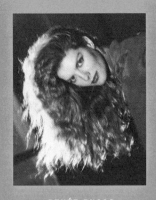

RENÉE RUSSO
ACTRESS

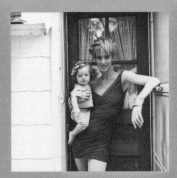

BONNIE BERMAN
FAMILY

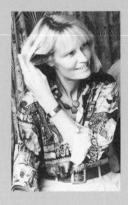

GUNILLA LINDBLAD
STORE OWNER

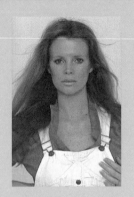

KIM BASSINGER
ACTRESS

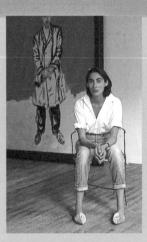

ANH DUONG
PAINTER

ELLEN VON UNWERTH
PHOTOGRAPHER

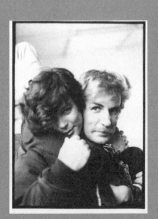

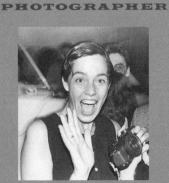

WALLIS FRANKEN + CLAUDE MONTANA
MUSE

LISA LOVE
EDITOR

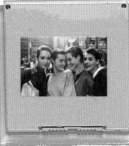
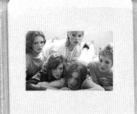
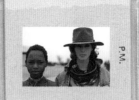

P.M.

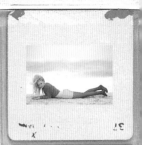

X

P.M.

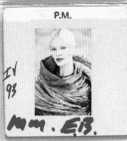

IV
93

mm . E.B.

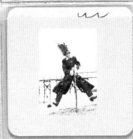

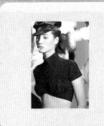

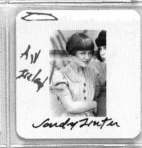

Arr
Iselaf

Sandy Linter

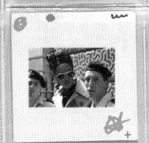

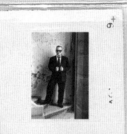

9

Vogue Br 1442

ARTHUR ELGORT

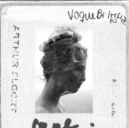

seve .

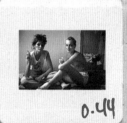

0.44

P.M.

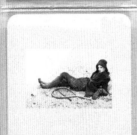

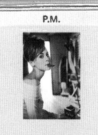

26

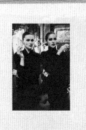

MAY 86 11

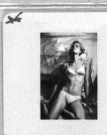

IV

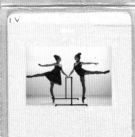

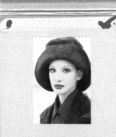

earls Linda

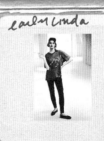

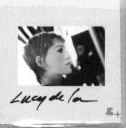

Lucy de la

S-+

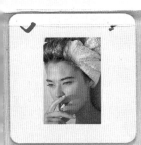
✓

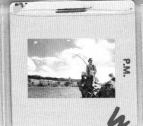
P.M.

4

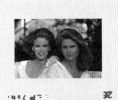
1466 d7

32

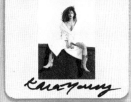
Kara Young

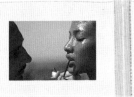

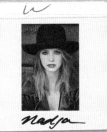
Nadja

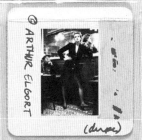
@ ARTHUR ELGORT
(dupe)

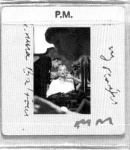
P.M.

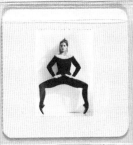
Nicole
Beech
T legs

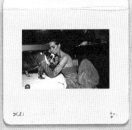

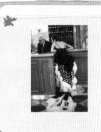

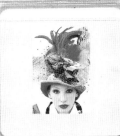
@ ARTHUR ELGORT

J & G

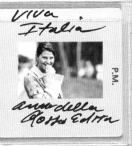
VIVA
Italia
P.M.
ann della
Rossa Editta

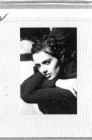

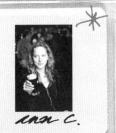
ann C.

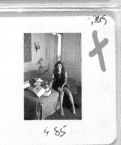
485

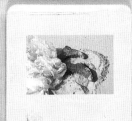

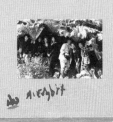
Alexbrit

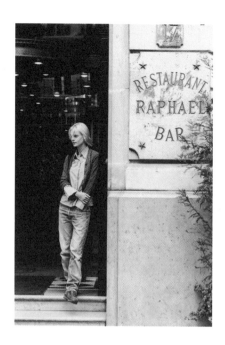

DON'T CANCEL A BOOKING ONCE YOU'VE SAID YES

MANAGE YOUR OWN MONEY

LEARN TO ACT LIKE SOMEONE ELSE, BUT ALSO BE YOURSELF

BE ON TIME

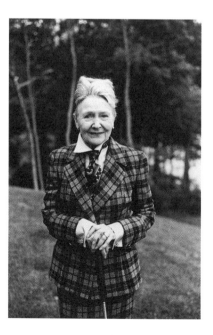

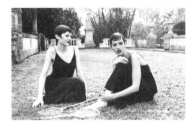

Don't be tense

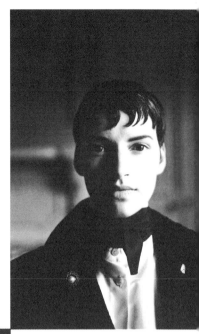

**DON'T
TALK
ON THE
PHONE
TOO
LONG**

BRING MUSIC TO THE SHOOT THAT YOU LIKE–JUST IN CASE

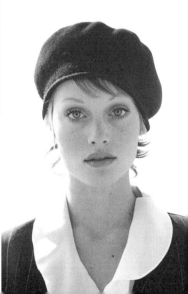

DON'T BE LAZY!

MODELS HAVE TO PRACTICE TOO,

IT'S A REAL JOB

**Line
up
some
nice
vacations
that
you
look
forward
to.
Late
December
and
August
are
good
times**

SIT, STAND, JUMP, LAUGH, CRY, RUNAWAY

LOOK AT THE CLOTHES. LOTS OF TIMES YOU WON'T LIKE THEM. HOW CAN YOU MAKE THEM WORK ? -

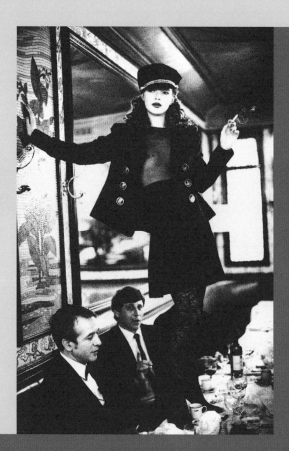

Look at yourself in the mirror once in a while

PRACTICE WALKING IN ALL KINDS OF SHOES

DON'T COMPLAIN!